HANDS-ON GUIDE TO
CLINICAL PHARMACOLOGY

D1078691

This book is dedicated to our families

HANDS-ON GUIDE TO CLINICAL PHARMACOLOGY

Sukhdev Chatu
Alexander Milson
Christopher Tofield

Final year medical students
St Bartholomew's and the Royal London Hospital School of
    Medicine and Dentistry
University of London

College adviser
Professor Nigel Benjamin
Professor of Clinical Pharmacology
St Bartholomew's and the Royal London Hospital School of
    Medicine and Dentistry
University of London

**Blackwell
Science**

© 2000 by
Blackwell Science Ltd
Editorial Offices:
Osney Mead, Oxford OX2 0EL
25 John Street, London
    WC1N 2BL
23 Ainslie Place, Edinburgh
    EH3 6AJ
350 Main Street, Malden
    MA 02148 5018, USA
54 University Street, Carlton
    Victoria 3053, Australia
10, rue Casimir Delavigne
    75006 Paris, France

Other Editorial Offices:
Blackwell Wissenschafts-Verlag
    GmbH
Kurfürstendamm 57
10707 Berlin, Germany

Blackwell Science KK
MG Kodenmacho Building
7–10 Kodenmacho Nihombashi
Chuo-ku, Tokyo 104, Japan

First published 2000
Reprinted 2001

Set by Graphicraft Limited,
Hong Kong

Printed and bound at
the Alden Press, Oxford
and Northampton

The Blackwell Science logo is a
trade mark of Blackwell Science
Ltd, registered at the United
Kingdom Trade Marks Registry

DISTRIBUTORS
Marston Book Services Ltd
PO Box 269
Abingdon, Oxon OX14 4YN
(Orders: Tel: 01235 465500
         Fax: 01235 465555)

The Americas
Blackwell Publishing
c/o AIDC
PO Box 20
50 Winter Sport Lane
Williston, VT 05495 0020
(Orders: Tel: 800 216 2522
         Fax: 802 864 7626)

Australia
Blackwell Science Pty Ltd
54 University Street
Carlton, Victoria 3053
(Orders: Tel: 3 9347 0300
         Fax: 3 9347 5001)

A catalogue record for this title is
available from the British Library

ISBN 0-632-05518-9

Library of Congress
Cataloging-in-publication Data
Chatu, Sukhdev
    Hands-on guide to clinical
pharmacology / Sukhdev
Chatu, Alexander Milson,
Christopher Tofield.
        p. ; cm.
    Includes bibliographical
references and index.
ISBN 0-632-05518-9
    1. Clinical pharmacology—
Handbooks, manuals, etc,
I. Milson, Alexander. II.
Tofield, Christopher. III. Title.
    [DNLM: 1. Drug Therapy
—methods—Handbooks.
2. Pharmacology, Clinical—
methods—Handbooks.
QV 39 C495h 2000
RM301.28.C48 2000
615'.—dc21   99–08908

For further information on
Blackwell Science, visit our website:
www.medirect.com

CONTENTS

PREFACE

- This new book in pharmacology should fill the gap that exists between the voluminous textbooks, too comprehensive and detailed for everyday use, and the scattered and fragmented information on individual drugs available from other various sources. It has a two-fold purpose:
  1 To provide a study aid for all students involved in the study of clinical pharmacology.
  2 To serve as a practical reference on the wards.
- This book contains information on 105 drugs, which you are most likely to encounter on the hospital wards or during your course of study. Doses have purposely been omitted (except for anaphylactic shock) since these are best obtained from an appropriate local or national formulary.
- We hope that finding information is facilitated by the simple text layout. Sections containing both treatment regimens of common conditions and detailed information on the relevant drugs will help the reader obtain a better understanding of current therapeutic management.
- The adverse effects and interactions shown in this book are not exhaustive. We have selected important interactions where appropriate, and emboldened those which are particularly likely to have important clinical consequences. For a full list of interactions, the *British National Formulary* should be consulted.
- 'Related drugs' refers to those which are of the same class and have similar pharmacological properties.
- This book has been designed as a quick reference and learning tool. It is not intended to provide an exhaustive account of clinical pharmacology. Other more detailed texts should be consulted if more information is required.
- We would welcome and value any reader feedback. Let us know how you think this approach could be improved by e-mailing us at authors@blacksci.co.uk.

ACKNOWLEDGEMENTS

We would like to thank the following teaching staff at our college for their advice and for providing up-to-date information:

Professor N. Benjamin, Professor of Clinical Pharmacology
Professor M. Caulfield, Professor of Clinical Pharmacology

Dr S. Aylwin, Lecturer in Endocrinology
Dr O. C. Cockerell, Senior Lecturer and Honorary Consultant in Neurology
Dr T. Crake, Consultant in Cardiology
Dr P. J. Flynn, Senior Lecturer and Honorary Consultant in Anaesthetics
Professor J. G. Grudzinskas, Professor of Obstetrics and Gynaecology
Dr A. Jawad, Senior Lecturer and Honorary Consultant in Rheumatology
Professor D. J. Jeffries, Professor of Virology
Dr S. O'Byrne, Lecturer in Clinical Pharmacology
Dr J. M. Parkin, Senior Lecturer and Consultant in Clinical Immunology
Dr A. Reinhardt, Specialist Registrar in Respiratory Medicine
Dr M. Salter, Consultant in Psychiatry
Professor M. Swash, Professor of Neurology
Professor P. Swain, Professor of Gastroenterology

ABBREVIATIONS

ACE inhibitor	Angiotensin-converting enzyme inhibitor
ADH	Antidiuretic hormone
AIDS	Acquired immunodeficiency syndrome
AMP	Adenosine monophosphate
5-ASA	5-aminosalicylic acid
ATP	Adenosine triphosphate
AV	Atrioventricular
BCG	Bacille Calmette–Guérin
BDZ	Benzodiazepine
BMI	Body mass index
CABG	Coronary artery bypass grafting
CHD	Coronary heart disease
CMV	Cytomegalovirus
CNS	Central nervous system
COC	Combined oral contraceptive
COPD	Chronic obstructive pulmonary disease
COX	Cyclo-oxygenase
CPR	Cardio-pulmonary resuscitation
CTG	Cardiotocography
DC shock	Direct current shock
DMARD	Disease-modifying antirheumatic drug
DNA	Deoxyribonucleic acid
DT	Diphtheria, tetanus
DTP	Diphtheria, tetanus, pertussis
EBV	Epstein–Barr virus
ECG	Electrocardiogram
ENT	Ear, nose and throat
FBC	Full blood count
FSH	Follicle-stimulating hormone
GABA	Gamma amino butyric acid
GI	Gastrointestinal
GTN	Glyceryl trinitrate
H_2 antagonist	Histamine 2 antagonist
Hb	Haemoglobin
HDL	High density lipoprotein
Hib	*Haemophilus influenzae* type b
HIV	Human immunodeficiency virus
HMG CoA	3-hydroxy 3-methylglutaryl co-enzyme A
HRT	Hormone replacement therapy
5-HT	5-hydroxytryptamine
IM	Intramuscular
INR	International normalized ratio

ISA	Intrinsic sympathomimetic activity
ITU	Intensive therapy unit
IUCD	Intrauterine contraceptive device
IUGR	Intrauterine growth restriction
IV	Intravenous
LDL	Low density lipoprotein
LFT	Liver function test
MAO	Monoamine oxidase
MAOI	Monoamine oxidase inhibitor
MI	Myocardial infarction
MMR	Mumps, measles, rubella
MRSA	Methicillin-resistant *Staphylococcus aureus*
NSAID	Non-steroidal anti-inflammatory drug
PE	Pulmonary embolus
PID	Pelvic inflammatory disease
POP	Progestogen-only pill
RNA	Ribonucleic acid
rt-PA	Recombinant tissue plasminogen activator
SA	Sinoatrial
SLE	Systemic lupus erythematosus
SSRI	Selective serotonin re-uptake inhibitor
TB	Tuberculosis
TCA	Tricyclic antidepressant
TG	Triglyceride
TSH	Thyroid-stimulating hormone
U&E	Urea and electrolytes
UTI	Urinary tract infection
VLDL	Very low density lipoprotein

INTRODUCTION

During the course of our studies at St Bartholomew's and the Royal London Hospital School of Medicine and Dentistry we realized that we were in need of a practical yet concise set of notes to revise clinical pharmacology.

What had initially been a collated set of revision notes was subsequently turned into structured and publishable material. We owe special thanks to our college adviser Professor Nigel Benjamin for his unfailing support, to Professor Mark Caulfield for his inspiration and sound advice, and to our families for their backing. We would also like to thank all the other teaching staff at our college who advised us and Dr Michael Stein at Blackwell Science for his faith in us.

S. Chatu
A. Milson
C. Tofield

CARDIOVASCULAR SYSTEM

This chapter provides an account of the management of common cardiovascular conditions, many of which have a high morbidity and mortality rate. Important relevant drugs are included.

MYOCARDIAL INFARCTION
- Sit the patient up (to ease breathing and reduce venous return to the heart)
- Give 60% oxygen through face mask (24% in COPD)
- Attach cardiac monitor and perform 12-lead ECG
- Take blood for FBC, U&E, cardiac enzymes and cholesterol
- Pain relief: give IV diamorphine with IV anti-emetic (e.g. metoclopramide)
- Limit infarct size:
  - Give aspirin (chewed or dissolved in water)
  - Give thrombolytic therapy if not contraindicated, preferably within 12 hours following MI (streptokinase or rt-PA)
- Admit to coronary care unit

POST-MYOCARDIAL INFARCTION
- Heparin infusion may be given to maintain vessel patency (of value only if given with rt-PA)
- If pain continues IV nitrates (e.g. GTN) can be given
- Look for and treat any complications:
  - Tachydysrhythmias—anti-arrhythmic drugs, DC shock or overdrive pacing
  - Bradydysrhythmias—IV atropine, pacing
  - Left ventricular failure with pulmonary oedema—IV furosemide followed by long-term ACE inhibitor
  - Cardiogenic shock—IV dopamine and IV dobutamine
  - Ventricular septal rupture/rupture of papillary muscle—urgent surgery
- Prevention of reinfarction:
  - Daily aspirin for life and a β blocker (e.g. atenolol) for a minimum of 2–3 years
  - Long term ACE inhibitor (e.g. captopril) if there is any left ventricular dysfunction
  - Add a statin (e.g. simvastatin) if cholesterol > 4.8 mmol/L
  - Alter modifiable risk factors (smoking, obesity, hyperlipidaemia, hypertension, diabetes mellitus)
- Consider coronary angioplasty or coronary bypass surgery on the basis of a coronary angiogram if necessary
- Advise no driving for 1 month and no work for 2 months

STABLE ANGINA
• Alter modifiable risk factors (smoking, hypertension, hyper-lipidaemia, diabetes mellitus, obesity, diet, lack of exercise)
• First line therapy: sublingual GTN spray/tablet or skin patch for acute attacks
• Maintenance therapy: β blocker (e.g. atenolol)
• If still symptomatic, add a calcium channel blocker or a long-acting oral nitrate (isosorbide mononitrate or isosorbide dinitrate)
• If still symptomatic, give maintenance triple therapy (β blocker, calcium channel blocker and a long-acting nitrate) + GTN for acute attacks
• *Note*: Do not give β blockers with verapamil due to serious interactions
• Nicorandil, a K^+ channel activator with vasodilator properties, is being increasingly used in the management of angina
• Last resort is coronary angioplasty or coronary bypass surgery

UNSTABLE ANGINA
• Give regular oral aspirin to prevent infarction
• Give IV heparin (to prevent infarction in acute attack)
• Give IV nitrates (e.g. GTN), an oral β blocker and an oral calcium channel blocker (e.g. nifedipine)
• If still symptomatic, consider emergency coronary angioplasty or coronary bypass surgery

ACUTE HEART FAILURE
• Sit the patient up
• Give 60% oxygen through face mask (24% in COPD)
• Give IV furosemide
• Give IV diamorphine (unless hepatic failure or COPD/asthma present) with IV anti-emetic (e.g. metoclopramide)
• If no improvement consider IV GTN
• In cardiogenic shock (signified by falling blood pressure) consider positive inotropes (dopamine, dobutamine)

CHRONIC HEART FAILURE
• Reduce salt intake and alter modifiable risk factors (e.g. smoking, obesity)
• Treat any underlying cause (e.g. hypertension, valvular heart disease)
• If still symptomatic give a loop diuretic (e.g. furosemide) with a thiazide diuretic (e.g. bendrofluazide)
• If still symptomatic add an ACE inhibitor (e.g. captopril)
• If still no improvement consider digoxin
• Venodilators, oral nitrates and arterial dilators can also be used
• β blocker + spironolactone (a potassium-sparing diuretic) have been shown to be of benefit in chronic heart failure

SUPRAVENTRICULAR DYSRHYTHMIAS
Acute atrial fibrillation (AF)
- Administer warfarin for 1 month, then give DC shock under general anaesthetic to revert to sinus rhythm (only if no structural heart lesions are present)
- Alternatively, give oral amiodarone or sotalol to revert to and maintain sinus rhythm
- If still symptomatic, treat as chronic AF

Chronic atrial fibrillation
- Regular oral digoxin
- If digoxin alone is not effective, add a β blocker or a calcium channel blocker (verapamil, diltiazem)
- Anticoagulation with warfarin is important to prevent emboli causing stroke or organ ischaemia (if contraindicated, give aspirin)

Atrial flutter
- Treat as for acute atrial fibrillation
- In chronic atrial flutter maintain on oral digoxin

Supraventricular tachycardia (SVT)
- Perform vagal manoeuvres (e.g. carotid sinus massage, immersion of the face in cold water)
- If this fails, give IV adenosine or IV verapamil
- If this fails, give synchronized DC shock
- In chronic SVT amiodarone can be used

VENTRICULAR DYSRHYTHMIAS
Ventricular fibrillation (VF, pulseless VT)
- Consult European Resuscitation Council guidelines

Ventricular tachycardia with a pulse (VT)
- Give IV lidocaine
- If this fails, give IV amiodarone or flecainide
- Proceed to synchronized DC shock in case of circulatory collapse or if there is no response with anti-arrhythmic drugs
- If still symptomatic, consider implantable defibrillator and electrical ablation of abnormal foci

HYPERTENSION
- Alter modifiable risk factors (e.g. smoking, obesity, alcohol, salt intake)
- Rule out secondary causes of hypertension (e.g. renal artery stenosis, Cushing's disease, coarctation of the aorta)
- The following classes of antihypertensives are used in various combinations (tailored to the individual):
  1 Thiazide diuretics (e.g. bendrofluazide)
  2 β blockers (e.g. atenolol)
  3 Calcium channel blockers (e.g. nifedipine)

4 ACE inhibitors (e.g. captopril)
5 Angiotensin II receptor antagonists (e.g. losartan)
6 α blockers (e.g. doxazosin)
7 Centrally acting agents (e.g. methyldopa, moxonidine)

PULMONARY EMBOLISM
- Gain IV access with a heparinized cannula
- Attach cardiac monitor
- Give 60% oxygen through face mask
- Give a NSAID for pleuritic pain
- For continuing pain, consider IV diamorphine + IV anti-emetic (e.g. metoclopramide)
- Give an IV heparin loading dose followed by heparin infusion
- Start oral warfarin at the same time as heparin and continue warfarin for 6 months (discontinue heparin when INR reaches therapeutic range)
- Consider thrombolytic therapy (e.g. streptokinase) in cases of a large pulmonary embolism

DEEP VEIN THROMBOSIS
- Give IV or low molecular weight subcutaneous heparin with oral warfarin
- Discontinue heparin when INR reaches therapeutic range
- For long term anticoagulation: continue warfarin for a minimum of 3–6 months
- Consider thrombolytic therapy (e.g. streptokinase) in cases of large thrombi

ANAPHYLACTIC SHOCK
- Give 1 mg (1 mL of 1 : 1000) epinephrine IM
- Give oxygen through face mask
- Gain IV access
- Give 10 mg of an antihistamine IV (chlorpheniramine)
- Give 100 mg hydrocortisone IV
- Consider IV aminophylline if bronchospasm present
- Administer IV fluids if required to maintain blood pressure
- Repeat epinephrine every 10 min if no improvement
- If still no improvement, consider intubation and mechanical ventilation

HYPERLIPIDAEMIA
- Modify diet (increase unsaturated and decrease saturated fats)
- Treat any underlying causes of hyperlipidaemia: hypothyroidism, diabetes mellitus, chronic alcohol intake, drugs (e.g. thiazide diuretics, β blockers)

- Hypercholesterolaemia: treat with a HMG CoA reductase inhibitor (e.g. simvastatin) if cholesterol levels > 5.5 mmol/L (or if > 4.8 mmol/L in patients with previous MI)
- Bile acid resins (e.g. cholestyramine) can also be used to decrease cholesterol levels
- In mixed hyperlipidaemia (high cholesterol and high triglycerides), or in hypertriglyceridaemia, fibrates can be given (e.g. bezafibrate)

Drug classes

ACE INHIBITORS
- Many types of ACE inhibitors exist, all of which have similar properties. Captopril, lisinopril and enalapril are commonly used.

Indications
- Hypertension
- Heart failure
- Post-myocardial infarction
- Diabetic nephropathy

Note
- ACE inhibitors are generally well-tolerated and have been shown to reduce mortality and morbidity in patients with heart failure (they are thought to prevent enlargement of the left ventricle).
- Angiotensin II receptor antagonists, such as losartan, have similar effects but their usefulness in heart failure has not been established.

β BLOCKERS
- There are two types of β receptors: β_1 and β_2
- β_1 receptors are found in the heart
- Most other β receptors are β_2 receptors and are found in the periphery

Types of β blockers
1 Selective (blocking β_1 receptors): atenolol, bisoprolol and metoprolol
2 Non-selective (blocking both β_1 and β_2 receptors): nadolol, propranolol and timolol
- *Note*: Selective β_1 blockers may also block β_2 receptors to some extent, especially in high doses
- β blockers can be either water-soluble, which are excreted renally unchanged (atenolol, nadolol, sotalol), or lipid-soluble, which are metabolized by the liver prior to excretion (metoprolol, propranolol)

- Some act as partial agonists (i.e. have ISA properties) such as oxprenolol and pindolol. They can block and stimulate β receptors at the same time. This results in less bradycardia and less peripheral vasoconstriction than with other β blockers.
- Labetolol and carvedilol block both α and β receptors

Indications
- Hypertension
- Angina
- Supraventricular dysrhythmias
- Secondary prophylaxis in myocardial infarction
- Non-selective β blockers can further be used in:
  - Thyrotoxicosis (to control symptoms)
  - Prophylaxis of migraine
  - Glaucoma
  - Anxiety (to prevent palpitations, tremor and tachycardia)

Effects
- β blockers can block β receptors in the heart, kidney, airways, skeletal muscle and blood vessels and can therefore cause the following effects:
  - β_1 receptor blockade—decreased force of myocardial contraction and heart rate
  - β_2 receptor blockade in the kidneys—decreased renin production and lowered blood pressure
  - β_2 receptor blockade in skeletal muscle—tiredness
  - β_2 receptor blockade in the airways—bronchospasm
  - β_2 receptor blockade in blood vessels—peripheral vasoconstriction (i.e. cold extremities)
- Lipid-soluble β blockers cross the blood–brain barrier and can cause sleep disturbance and nightmares (this also applies to water-soluble β blockers, but to a lesser extent)

CALCIUM CHANNEL BLOCKERS
Types of calcium channel blockers
1 Dihydropyridines: nifedipine, amlodipine, nicardipine, isradepine
2 Phenylalkalamines: verapamil
3 Benzothiapines: diltiazem

Indications
- Hypertension
- Angina (dihydropyridines are used with a β blocker; verapamil or diltiazem on their own)
- Dysrhythmias (verapamil or diltiazem)

Mechanism of action
- All calcium channel blockers act on L-type calcium channels at different sites:
  - Myocardium

- The conducting system of the heart
- Vascular smooth muscle.

Verapamil and diltiazem
- Verapamil and diltiazem act both on the heart and peripheral blood vessels. They decrease the heart rate, the force of contraction and have anti-arrhythmic properties. They also cause peripheral vasodilatation and dilatation of coronary arteries.
- Verapamil and diltiazem must be used with extreme caution with β blockers due to hazardous interactions such as asystole and AV node block

Dihydropyridines
- Dihydropyridines act mainly on peripheral and coronary vasculature and are therefore used to treat angina (usually combined with a β blocker)
- Dihydropyridines can be used alone in the treatment of hypertension or can be safely combined with a β blocker
- Dihydropyridines have very few cardiac effects

DIURETICS
Types of diuretics
1 Thiazides: bendrofluazide
2 Loop diuretics: furosemide, bumetanide
3 Potassium-sparing: spironolactone, amiloride
4 Carbonic anhydrase inhibitors: acetazolamide, dorzolamide
5 Osmotic: mannitol

Indications
- Hypertension (thiazides)
- Chronic heart failure (loop diuretics, thiazides or in combination)
- Oedema (loop diuretics, thiazides or in combination)
- Glaucoma (acetazolamide, dorzolamide, mannitol)
- Raised intracranial pressure (mannitol)

Mechanism of action
- Diuretics generally act on the nephron in the kidney to increase sodium and water excretion.

Note
- Loop diuretics are the most effective diuretics, followed by thiazides.
- Potassium-sparing diuretics are weak and not normally used on their own. They are usually given with loop diuretics and thiazides to prevent hypokalaemia.
- Potassium-sparing diuretics should not normally be used with ACE inhibitors as dangerous hyperkalaemia may result.
- Loop and thiazide diuretics act synergistically and are effective in the treatment of resistant oedema.

Adenosine

Class: Anti-arrhythmic agent

Indications
- Supraventricular dysrhythmias

Mechanism of action
- Adenosine acts on the SA and AV nodes by binding to adenosine receptors in the conducting tissue of the heart. This slows conduction through the heart and causes a decrease in the heart rate.

Adverse effects
- *Common*: chest pain, bronchospasm, flushing, nausea (all transient, lasting < 1 min)
- *Rare*: severe bradycardia

Contraindications
- Asthma
- 2nd or 3rd degree heart block (unless pacemaker is *in situ*)
- Sick sinus syndrome

Interactions
- *Dipyridamole*: adenosine enhances and prolongs the anti-platelet effect of dipyridamole
- *Theophylline*: theophylline inhibits the action of adenosine by blocking adenosine receptors

Route of administration
- IV bolus

Note
- Prior to administration of adenosine the patient should be warned about the transient adverse effects such as chest pain, as they may cause great distress.
- Adenosine has a very short duration of action (about 8 seconds), therefore adverse effects are mostly short-lived.

Amiodarone

Class: Anti-arrhythmic agent

Indications
- Supraventricular dysrhythmias
- Ventricular dysrhythmias

Mechanism of action
- Amiodarone prolongs the refractory period in all parts of the conducting system of the heart. This decreases the speed of impulses moving through the heart.

Adverse effects
- *Common*: reversible corneal depositions (in long term use), photosensitive rash
- *Rare*: hypothyroidism or hyperthyroidism, pulmonary fibrosis, hepatitis, neurological symptoms (e.g. tremor, ataxia), peripheral neuropathy, grey skin colour

Contraindications
- Cardiac conduction defects (e.g. sick sinus syndrome)
- Thyroid disease
- Pregnancy
- Breast feeding
- Iodine allergy (as amiodarone contains iodine)

Interactions
- ***β blockers***: concomitant use of amiodarone and β blockers increases the risk of bradycardia, AV block and myocardial depression
- ***Digoxin***: amiodarone increases the plasma concentration of digoxin, thus increasing the risk of digoxin toxicity
- *Diltiazem, verapamil*: concomitant use of amiodarone with diltiazem or verapamil increases the risk of bradycardia, AV block and myocardial depression
- ***Disopyramide, quinidine, procainamide***: amiodarone has an additive effect with these drugs and, as they all increase the QT interval on the ECG, they should not be used together
- ***Phenytoin***: amiodarone inhibits the metabolism of phenytoin
- ***Warfarin***: amiodarone enhances the effect of warfarin by inhibiting its metabolism

Route of administration
- Oral, IV

Note
- Amiodarone has a half-life of about 36 days and so interactions can occur long after the drug has been stopped.
- Thyroid and liver functions should be monitored every 6 months whilst on treatment with amiodarone.
- Pulmonary function tests should be performed prior to and during treatment with amiodarone in order to detect any developing pulmonary fibrosis.

Atenolol

Class: β_1 blocker

Indications
- Hypertension
- Angina
- Supraventricular dysrhythmias
- Secondary prophylaxis of myocardial infarction
- Prophylaxis of migraine

Mechanism of action
- Atenolol reduces heart rate and force of myocardial contraction by acting on β_1 receptors in the heart. This results in decreased workload of the heart, hence its use in angina.
- Renin production by the kidney is also reduced by atenolol, which contributes to its antihypertensive effect.
- Atenolol decreases the effects of sympathetic activity on the heart with a resulting decrease in conduction and in action potential initiation. Hence its antiarrhythmic effect.

Adverse effects
- *Common*: lethargy (usually ceases after long term use), bradycardia and AV block, hypotension, cold peripheries
- *Rare*: bronchospasm, worsened or precipitated heart failure, nightmares

Contraindications
- Asthma
- Heart failure
- 2nd and 3rd degree heart block
- Bradycardia
- COPD
- Phaeochromocytoma

Interactions
- *Diltiazem*: concomitant use of diltiazem and atenolol increases the risk of bradycardia and AV block
- *Insulin and oral hypoglycaemics*: β blockers mask the symptoms of hypoglycaemia caused by oral hypoglycaemics or insulin
- *Verapamil*: the risk of heart failure, bradycardia and AV block is increased if atenolol is given with verapamil

Route of administration
- Oral, IV

Note
- Atenolol is selective for β_1 receptors, but at high doses it can also block β_2 receptors thus causing bronchospasm.
- Abrupt withdrawal of atenolol may worsen angina.

Related drugs
- Bisoprolol, metoprolol (β_1 blockers); nadolol, propranolol ($\beta_1 + \beta_2$ blockers)

Atropine

Class: Muscarinic antagonist

Indications
- Cardio-pulmonary resuscitation
- Bradycardia
- Organophosphorus poisoning
- To paralyse the ciliary muscle (allowing measurement of the refractive error in children)
- Irritable bowel syndrome

Mechanism of action
- Atropine decreases the activity of the parasympathetic nervous system by blocking the action of acetylcholine on muscarinic receptors. This leads to pupillary dilatation, bronchodilatation, increase in heart rate and decreased secretions from sweat, salivary and bronchial glands. It also reduces gut motility and secretions.

Adverse effects
- *Common*: dry mouth, blurred vision, constipation
- *Rare*: confusion (especially in the elderly), palpitations, irritation of the eye (when given as eye drops), acute urinary retention

Contraindications
- Prostatic hypertrophy
- Closed-angle glaucoma
- Paralytic ileus
- Myasthenia gravis
- Pyloric stenosis

Interactions
- *Antidepressants (TCAs, MAOIs)*: these can potentiate anticholinergic adverse effects of atropine

Route of administration
- Oral (rarely used for irritable bowel syndrome), IV (bradycardia, CPR), IM (organophosphorus poisoning), eye drops (to paralyse the ciliary muscle)

Note
- Atropine can be used to reverse the adverse effects of neostigmine (e.g. bradycardia). In this case it is given IV.

Bendrofluazide

Class: Thiazide diuretic

Indications
- Hypertension
- Heart failure
- Oedema (secondary to liver disease, nephrotic syndrome or low protein diet)
- Prophylaxis of calcium-containing renal stones

Mechanism of action
- Bendrofluazide acts on the proximal part of the distal tubule in the nephron where it inhibits Na^+ and Cl^- reabsorption. This leads to increased excretion of Na^+, Cl^- and water, which stimulates potassium excretion further down in the distal tubule. All these events lead to hypokalaemia, hyponatraemia and a decrease in fluid volume.
- Reduced fluid volume causes an initial decrease in cardiac output (hence initial anti-hypertensive effect), but a reduction in peripheral resistance is responsible for lowering blood pressure in the long term.

Adverse effects
- *Common*: hypokalaemia, dehydration, postural hypotension
- *Rare*: impotence, lethargy, hyperuricaemia, hyperglycaemia, hyperlipidaemia, hypercalcaemia, thrombocytopenia, hyponatraemia

Contraindications
- Hypokalaemia, hyponatraemia, hypercalcaemia
- Severe hepatic and renal impairment
- Gout

Interactions
- *Digoxin*: hypokalaemia caused by bendrofluazide potentiates the effects of digoxin, thus increasing the risk of dysrhythmias
- *Lithium*: bendrofluazide increases the plasma concentration of lithium

Route of administration
- Oral

Note
- Low doses of bendrofluazide cause minimal biochemical disturbance and are fully effective at lowering blood pressure. Higher doses do not decrease blood pressure any further, but make adverse biochemical effects more likely.
- Prolonged use at high doses may lead to hypokalaemia, which can cause cardiac arrest (hence potassium levels must be monitored). If high doses are prescribed, it is recommended to combine bendrofluazide with either potassium supplements, a potassium-sparing diuretic (e.g. amiloride) or an ACE inhibitor.

Related drugs
- Chlorothiazide, chlorthalidone, hydrochlorothiazide

Bezafibrate

Class: Fibrate

Indications
- Hyperlipidaemia

Mechanism of action
- Bezafibrate reduces triglyceride levels by stimulating the enzyme lipoprotein lipase, which converts triglycerides into fatty acids and glycerol.
- Bezafibrate also reduces cholesterol levels (to a lesser extent) by reducing cholesterol production in the liver. It decreases circulating LDL levels and also increases the levels of beneficial HDL.

Adverse effects
- *Common*: nausea, abdominal discomfort, headache
- *Rare*: myositis syndrome (muscle pain, stiffness, weakness), impotence, rash, pruritus

Contraindications
- Renal impairment (risk of myositis syndrome)
- Hepatic impairment
- Hypoalbuminaemia
- Pregnancy
- Breast feeding
- Gallbladder disease

Interactions
- *HMG CoA reductase inhibitors*: concomitant use of bezafibrate and HMG CoA reductase inhibitors increases the risk of myositis syndrome
- *Warfarin*: bezafibrate potentiates the anticoagulant effect of warfarin by displacing it from plasma protein binding sites

Route of administration
- Oral

Note
- Drug treatment of hyperlipidaemia is recommended when patients fail to respond to dietary measures.
- It has been shown that fibrates are less effective than statins in the prevention of cardiovascular events (e.g. myocardial infarction).

Related drugs
- Ciprofibrate, fenofibrate, gemfibrozil

Captopril

Class: Angiotensin-converting enzyme inhibitor

Indications
- Hypertension
- Heart failure
- Post-myocardial infarction
- Diabetic nephropathy

Mechanism of action
- Captopril inhibits ACE leading to decreased synthesis of angiotensin II and to accumulation of bradykinin:
  - Angiotensin II causes peripheral vasoconstriction and stimulates aldosterone release, causing K^+ excretion and retention of Na^+ and water. Decreased angiotensin II levels thus reduce peripheral resistance and fluid overload. This enhances ventricular emptying and improves cardiac function.
  - Accumulation of bradykinin leads to peripheral vasodilatation.

Adverse effects
- *Common*: postural hypotension, dry cough, rash
- *Rare*: hyperkalaemia, worsening of renal function (in those with underlying renal ischaemia or severe heart failure), angioneurotic oedema, haematological toxicity (e.g. neutropenia, agranulocytosis)

Contraindications
- Renal vascular disease (e.g. renal artery stenosis)
- Pregnancy
- Aortic stenosis
- Porphyria

Interactions
- *Diuretics*: pronounced hypotension is more likely if captopril is used in conjunction with diuretics
- *Lithium*: captopril increases the plasma concentration of lithium by reducing its excretion
- *NSAIDs*: NSAIDs increase the risk of renal impairment
- *Potassium-sparing diuretics*: concomitant use of captopril and potassium-sparing diuretics increases the risk of hyperkalaemia, especially in patients with renal impairment

Route of administration
- Oral

Note
- Microalbuminuria is an early sign of nephropathy in diabetics. There is evidence that ACE inhibitors reduce the risk of further renal deterioration.
- The patient should be advised to take the first dose just before bed time to prevent first-dose hypotension.
- ACE inhibitors improve exercise tolerance and symptoms in heart failure. They also prolong life expectancy in these patients.

Related drugs
- Cilazapril, enalapril, fosinopril, lisinopril

Digoxin

Class: Cardiac glycoside

Indications
- Supraventricular dysrhythmias
- Heart failure

Mechanism of action
- The primary action of digoxin on the heart is to inhibit the Na^+/K^+ ATP pump. This increases intracellular Na^+ concentration, which in turn inhibits the Na^+/Ca^{2+} exchanger and hence the amount of calcium pumped out of the cell. These events lead to increased intracellular calcium in myocardial cells which increases the force of myocardial contraction.
- Digoxin slows the heart rate by increasing vagal activity. It also slows conduction through the AV node (hence its use in dysrhythmias).

Adverse effects
- *Common*: nausea, vomiting, anorexia, diarrhoea, digoxin toxicity in overdose (heart block, dysrhythmias), visual disturbances (e.g. yellow vision)
- *Rare*: confusion, hallucinations

Contraindications
- Complete heart block
- Hypertrophic obstructive cardiomyopathy
- Wolff–Parkinson–White syndrome

Interactions
- ***Amiodarone, propafenone, quinidine***: these anti-arrhythmic drugs increase the risk of digoxin toxicity
- ***Calcium channel blockers (diltiazem, nicardipine, verapamil)***: these increase the risk of digoxin toxicity
- ***Diuretics (loop and thiazide)***: hypokalaemia caused by diuretics can enhance the effects of digoxin, thus increasing the risk of toxicity (dysrhythmias, heart block)

Route of administration
- Oral, IV (for emergency loading dose)

Note
- In heart failure, digoxin does not reduce mortality but improves symptoms and reduces the frequency of hospital admissions at the expense of possible digoxin toxicity.
- Digoxin has a narrow therapeutic window and therefore requires therapeutic drug monitoring. Potassium levels should also be monitored regularly.
- The risk of digoxin toxicity is greater in hypokalaemia, hypercalcaemia and hypothyroidism.
- Patients receiving digoxin and potassium-losing diuretics may require potassium supplements or a potassium-sparing diuretic.

Related drugs
- Digitoxin

Diltiazem

Class: Calcium channel blocker

Indications
- Prophylaxis and treatment of angina
- Hypertension
- Cardiac dysrhythmias

Mechanism of action
- Diltiazem inhibits the influx of calcium into vascular smooth muscle and myocardium by binding to the L-type calcium channels. This results in:
  1 relaxation of vascular smooth muscle with subsequent decrease in peripheral resistance and blood pressure;
  2 decreased myocardial contractility; and
  3 slowed conduction at the AV node and prolonged refractory period (hence anti-arrhythmic properties).
- Reduction in afterload, myocardial contractility and heart rate leads to reduced oxygen consumption, thereby relieving angina.

Adverse effects
- *Common*: headache, nausea, dizziness, hypotension, bradycardia, ankle swelling
- *Rare*: lethargy, rash

Contraindications
- Severe bradycardia
- 2nd and 3rd degree heart block
- Heart failure
- Pregnancy
- Breast feeding

Interactions
- *Anti-arrhythmics*: diltiazem may potentiate the myocardial depression caused by other anti-arrhythmic drugs
- *β blockers*: β blockers increase the risk of AV block and bradycardia with diltiazem
- *Cyclosporin*: diltiazem increases the plasma concentration of cyclosporin
- *Digoxin*: diltiazem increases the plasma concentration of digoxin
- *Theophylline*: diltiazem enhances the effects of theophylline

Route of administration
- Oral

Note
- Diltiazem can be used in patients with coronary artery spasm (Prinzmetal's angina).
- Diltiazem has the fewest adverse effects of all calcium channel blockers.
- It has a short half-life due to extensive first pass metabolism.

Related drugs
- Verapamil

Dobutamine

Class: Inotropic sympathomimetic

Indications
- Inotropic support in the following:
  - Acute severe heart failure
  - Cardiogenic shock
  - Cardiac surgery
  - Septic shock

Mechanism of action
- Dobutamine increases cardiac contractility with less effect on heart rate than dopamine. It works through stimulation of β_1 adrenoceptors in the heart.

Adverse effects
- *Common*: tachycardia
- *Rare*: ventricular dysrhythmias

Contraindications
- None
- Caution:
  - Severe hypotension
  - Tachycardia
  - Ischaemic cardiac pain

Interactions
- None

Route of administration
- IV infusion

Note
- Dobutamine does not reduce renal perfusion and for this reason is preferred to α agonists in the treatment of shock.
- Dobutamine is often combined with low dose dopamine in the treatment of cardiogenic shock.

Dopamine

Class: Inotropic sympathomimetic

Indications
- Cardiogenic shock following myocardial infarction
- Hypotension following cardiac surgery
- Acute severe heart failure
- Initiation of diuresis in chronic heart failure

Mechanism of action
- The actions of dopamine are dose-dependent.
  - In low doses (< 5 µg/kg/min), dopamine acts on dopamine receptors resulting in renal vasodilatation and improved renal perfusion.
  - In moderate doses (5–20 µg/kg/min), dopamine increases cardiac contractility and causes tachycardia by acting on cardiac β_1 adrenoceptors.
  - In high doses (> 20 µg/kg/min), dopamine causes vasoconstriction by acting on α adrenoceptors.

Adverse effects
- *Common*:
  - Low doses: nausea, vomiting
  - Moderate to high doses: tachycardia, ventricular ectopic beats, peripheral vasoconstriction, hypotension or hypertension

Contraindications
- Tachycardia
- Phaeochromocytoma

Interactions
- *MAOIs*: dopamine can cause a hypertensive crisis if given with MAOIs

Route of administration
- IV infusion

Note
- Moderate and high doses of dopamine must be administered through a central venous line.
- Blood pressure, heart rate and urine output must be monitored during treatment.
- Dopamine should not be infused into alkaline solutions as this would render it inactive.

Doxazosin

Class: α_1 blocker

Indications
- Hypertension
- Benign prostatic hyperplasia (BPH)

Mechanism of action
- Doxazosin inhibits α_1-mediated vasoconstriction, thus causing reduction in peripheral resistance with a subsequent fall in blood pressure.
- Doxazosin also relaxes smooth muscle in the internal urethral sphincter resulting in increased urinary outflow in BPH.

Adverse effects
- *Common*: postural hypotension, dizziness, headache, nausea, vomiting
- *Rare*: rhinitis, rash

Contraindications
- None
- Caution:
  - Hepatic impairment
  - Pregnancy
  - Breast feeding

Interactions
- *Antidepressants*: doxazosin enhances the hypotensive effect of antidepressants
- *β blockers*: doxazosin enhances the hypotensive effect of β blockers
- *Calcium channel blockers*: doxazosin enhances the hypotensive effect of calcium channel blockers
- *Diuretics:* doxazosin enhances the hypotensive effect of diuretics

Route of administration
- Oral

Note
- Long term therapy with doxazosin lowers plasma LDL, VLDL and triglyceride levels. It also increases HDL levels and is therefore considered beneficial in patients with coronary heart disease.

Related drugs
- Indoramin, prazosin, terazosin

Epinephrine (adrenaline)

Class: Sympathomimetic agent

Indications
- Anaphylactic shock
- Cardio-pulmonary resuscitation
- To prolong the effects of local anaesthetics
- Open-angle glaucoma

Mechanism of action
- Epinephrine has various effects due to stimulation of the sympathetic nervous system. It is a potent α and β receptor agonist.
  - α receptor stimulation causes vasoconstriction which prolongs the action of local anaesthetics by preventing their spread from the site of application.
  - β_1 receptor stimulation increases the heart rate and force of myocardial contraction. β_2 receptor stimulation results in vasodilatation, bronchodilatation and uterine relaxation.
- Epinephrine is useful in the treatment of anaphylactic shock as it raises blood pressure and causes bronchodilatation.
- Epinephrine is thought to decrease the production of aqueous humour and increase its outflow from the anterior chamber of the eye, hence its use in glaucoma.

Adverse effects
- *Common*: anxiety, restlessness, tremor, tachycardia, hypertension
- *Rare*: dysrhythmias, cerebral haemorrhage, pulmonary oedema (all in overdose)

Contraindications
- Closed-angle glaucoma
- Caution:
  - Coronary heart disease
  - Hyperthyroidism
  - Hypertension

Interactions
- *β blockers*: β blockers can cause severe hypertension if given with epinephrine
- *TCAs*: TCAs increase the risk of dysrhythmias and hypertension if given with epinephrine

Route of administration
- IM (anaphylactic shock), IV (CPR), eye drops (open-angle glaucoma), subcutaneous (with local anaesthetics)

Note
- Epinephrine is frequently administered with local anaesthetics (e.g. lidocaine) except in the fingers, toes and penis where prolonged vasoconstriction may result in gangrene.
- In CPR epinephrine can be given through an endotracheal tube if IV access is unobtainable. In this case the dose should be doubled.

Furosemide (frusemide)

Class: Loop diuretic

Indications
- Acute pulmonary oedema secondary to left ventricular failure
- Chronic heart failure
- Oliguria secondary to acute renal failure

Mechanism of action
- Furosemide inhibits reabsorption of Na^+, K^+ and water in the ascending limb of the loop of Henle by inhibiting the $Na^+/K^+/2Cl^-$ pump at this site. This leads to increased salt, water and potassium loss.

Adverse effects
- *Common*: postural hypotension, hypokalaemia, hyponatraemia, hyperuricaemia and gout
- *Rare*: bone marrow suppression, GI disturbance, reversible deafness (only in high doses or patients with renal failure)

Contraindications
- Renal impairment

Interactions
- ***Antibacterials***: furosemide increases the risk of ototoxicity associated with aminoglycosides, colistin and vancomycin, and increases the risk of renal toxicity associated with aminoglycosides
- ***Digoxin***: furosemide-induced hypokalaemia enhances the effects of digoxin, thus increasing the risk of digoxin-induced dysrhythmias
- ***Lithium***: furosemide decreases lithium excretion, leading to an increased risk of lithium toxicity

Route of administration
- Oral, IM, IV

Note
- Furosemide causes potassium loss. A potassium-sparing diuretic (e.g. amiloride), potassium supplements or an ACE inhibitor should be prescribed with it.
- Loop diuretics are more effective than thiazide diuretics.

Related drugs
- Bumetanide, torasemide

Glyceryl trinitrate

Class: Organic nitrate

Indications
- Angina
- Heart failure

Mechanism of action
- Glyceryl trinitrate (GTN) is metabolized into nitric oxide (NO) within vascular smooth muscle cells. This compound causes relaxation of vascular smooth muscle through activation of guanylyl cyclase. The result of this is vasodilatation of coronary arteries and systemic veins, with ensuing decrease in preload and improved oxygen supply to the myocardium.

Adverse effects
- *Common*: headache, dizziness, postural hypotension, flushing, tachycardia

Contraindications
- Hypotension
- Aortic stenosis
- Mitral stenosis
- Constrictive pericarditis
- Cardiac tamponade
- Hypertrophic obstructive cardiomyopathy (HOCM)
- Head trauma
- Cerebral haemorrhage
- Closed-angle glaucoma

Interactions
- *Sildenafil*: sildenafil enhances the hypotensive effect of GTN

Route of administration
- Sublingual, skin patch or skin ointment (all for angina), IV (for severe angina and acute heart failure)

Note
- Duration of action of GTN is roughly 30 min.
- Isosorbide dinitrate and isosorbide mononitrate are other commonly used nitrates. Their properties are similar to those of GTN but they can be taken orally and have a longer duration of action (several hours).
- Tolerance to long-acting nitrates (isosorbide dinitrate and isosorbide mononitrate) develops after as little as 24 hours of continued administration. Their effects thus become progressively weaker. This can be minimized by allowing drug-free periods of 8 hours.

Related drugs
- Isosorbide dinitrate, isosorbide mononitrate

Heparin

Class: Anticoagulant

Indications
- Prophylaxis and treatment of deep vein thrombosis
- Pulmonary embolism
- Unstable angina
- Myocardial infarction
- Acute occlusion of peripheral arteries
- Extracorporeal circuits (e.g. haemodialysis, cardio-pulmonary bypass)

Mechanism of action
- Heparin potentiates the action of antithrombin III which inactivates thrombin and other factors (especially Xa) involved in the clotting pathway. This inhibits thrombus formation.

Adverse effects
- *Common*: haemorrhage, thrombocytopenia
- *Rare*: osteoporosis or alopecia with long term use, skin necrosis, rash, anaphylaxis

Contraindications
- Haemorrhage
- Haemophilia
- Active peptic ulceration
- Thrombocytopenia
- Following major trauma
- Recent stroke
- Recent surgery
- Heparin hypersensitivity

Interactions
- *Aspirin*: aspirin increases the risk of haemorrhage if given with heparin

Route of administration
- IV, subcutaneous

Note
- Heparin has an immediate effect, which makes it suitable for use in acute thrombotic states.
- The effects of heparin can be reversed by IV protamine sulphate injection.
- Two types of heparin are available: unfractionated heparin and low molecular weight heparin. They are both of equal efficacy, but low molecular weight heparin has a longer duration of action (e.g. dalteparin).
- Treatment must be monitored by measuring the activated partial thromboplastin time (APTT), preferably on a daily basis. However, routine prophylactic treatment with low molecular weight heparin does not require monitoring.

Related drugs
- Certoparin, dalteparin, enoxaparin, tinzaparin (all are low molecular weight heparins)

Methyldopa

Class: Centrally acting antihypertensive agent

Indications
- Hypertension

Mechanism of action
- Methyldopa is converted to its active component, α-methylnorepinephrine, within adrenergic nerve endings. This compound stimulates α_2 adrenoceptors of the vasomotor centre in the medulla, causing reduced sympathetic outflow. Subsequently, this leads to vasodilatation and a fall in blood pressure.

Adverse effects
- *Common*: drowsiness, headache, postural hypotension, depression, impotence
- *Rare*: haemolytic anaemia, diarrhoea, rash, nasal congestion

Contraindications
- Depression
- Active hepatic disease
- Porphyria
- Phaeochromocytoma

Interactions
- *Anaesthetics*: anaesthetics enhance the hypotensive effect of methyldopa
- *Lithium*: concomitant use of methyldopa and lithium may cause neurotoxicity

Route of administration
- Oral, IV infusion

Note
- Methyldopa is commonly prescribed for hypertension in pregnancy. Research has shown that it has no adverse effects on the fetus.

Related drugs
- Clonidine, moxonidine

Nifedipine

Class: Calcium channel blocker

Indications
- Hypertension
- Prophylaxis and treatment of angina
- Raynaud's disease

Mechanism of action
- Nifedipine inhibits the influx of calcium into vascular smooth muscle (and, to a lesser extent, into myocardium) by binding to the L-type calcium channels, especially in arterioles. This results in relaxation of vascular smooth muscle with a subsequent decrease in peripheral resistance and blood pressure.
- Nifedipine dilates coronary arteries, which contributes to its anti-anginal effect.

Adverse effects
- *Common*: headache, flushing, ankle swelling, dizziness, hypotension
- *Rare*: worsening of angina, urinary frequency

Contraindications
- Malignant hypertension
- Cardiogenic shock
- Advanced aortic stenosis
- Porphyria
- Myocardial infarction in the previous one month

Interactions
- *Diltiazem*: diltiazem reduces the clearance of nifedipine, thus increasing its plasma concentration
- *Grapefruit juice*: grapefruit juice raises the plasma concentration of nifedipine and other dihydropyridines (except amlodipine)
- **Phenytoin**: nifedipine increases the plasma concentration of phenytoin
- *Rifampicin*: rifampicin increases the metabolism of nifedipine, thus decreasing its effects

Route of administration
- Oral

Note
- Nifedipine can be safely used in asthmatics, for whom β blockers are contraindicated.
- For best effect in severe angina, nifedipine should be combined with a β blocker.

Related drugs
- Amlodipine, felodipine, isradipine, lacidipine, lercanadipine, nicardipine, nimodipine, nisoldipine

Simvastatin

Class: HMG CoA reductase inhibitor

Indications
- Hypercholesterolaemia

Mechanism of action
- Simvastatin reversibly inhibits HMG CoA reductase, the rate-limiting enzyme in cholesterol synthesis by the liver. The liver responds by increasing expression of LDL receptors, which increases LDL uptake from the plasma. These actions reduce plasma cholesterol.
- Simvastatin causes a small decrease in the plasma concentration of triglycerides.

Adverse effects
- *Rare*: reversible myositis, GI disturbance, abdominal pain, headache, rash, fatigue, alopecia, altered liver function tests

Contraindications
- Liver disease
- Pregnancy
- Breast feeding
- Porphyria

Interactions
- *Cyclosporin*: cyclosporin increases the risk of myositis if given with simvastatin
- *Fibrates*: these increase the risk of myositis if given with simvastatin
- *Itraconazole and ketoconazole*: these increase the risk of myopathy if given with simvastatin
- **Warfarin**: simvastatin enhances the effect of warfarin

Route of administration
- Oral

Note
- Simvastatin has been shown to be effective in reducing cardiovascular events and mortality in patients with known or at high risk of cardiovascular disease. The optimum amount of cholesterol reduction is not yet established in the prevention of cardiovascular disease.
- Simvastatin should only be prescribed if the patient has not responded sufficiently to diet modification and after secondary causes of hyperlipidaemia have been ruled out (e.g. hypothyroidism, chronic alcohol abuse).
- Liver function tests should be carried out before and 3 months after starting therapy and regularly thereafter.
- The patient should be advised to immediately report unexplained muscle pain, tenderness or weakness.

Related drugs
- Atorvastatin, cerivastatin, fluvastatin, pravastatin

Streptokinase

Class: Fibrinolytic agent

Indications
- Acute myocardial infarction
- Thromboembolic events (e.g. pulmonary embolism, deep vein thrombosis, thrombosed arterio-venous shunts)

Mechanism of action
- Streptokinase binds to circulating plasminogen and forms an activator complex that converts plasminogen to plasmin. Plasmin then lyses the fibrin within the thrombus, thus dissolving it.

Adverse effects
- *Common*: hypotension, allergic reactions (e.g. rash, flushing)
- *Rare*: bleeding, anaphylaxis, Guillain–Barré syndrome

Contraindications
- Recent haemorrhage
- Bleeding disorders
- Recent trauma or surgery
- Aortic dissection
- Previous streptokinase treatment in the past year (due to remaining circulating antibodies to streptokinase)
- Severe hepatic impairment
- Acute pancreatitis
- Coma

Interactions
- ***Warfarin***: warfarin increases the risk of haemorrhage if given with streptokinase

Route of administration
- IV

Note
- Streptokinase is produced by β-haemolytic streptococci.
- The human body generates antibodies to streptokinase. If the patient has received streptokinase in the past year, alteplase (rt-PA) should be used instead. Alteplase is non-immunogenic.
- Fresh frozen plasma with tranexamic acid (antifibrinolytic agent) may be given if streptokinase treatment results in excessive bleeding.
- Streptokinase should be given within 12 hours of myocardial infarction. However, the greatest fibrinolytic effect is achieved if given within the first 3 hours.

Related drugs
- Alteplase (rt-PA), anistreplase, reteplase, urokinase

Verapamil

Class: Calcium channel blocker

Indications
- Hypertension
- Angina
- Supraventricular dysrhythmias

Mechanism of action
- Verapamil inhibits influx of calcium into vascular smooth muscle and myocardium by binding to the L-type calcium channels. This results in:

  1 relaxation of vascular smooth muscle with subsequent decrease in peripheral resistance and blood pressure;

  2 decreased myocardial contractility; and

  3 slowed conduction through the AV node and prolonged refractory period (hence anti-arrhythmic properties).
- Angina is relieved by reduction in afterload, heart rate and myocardial contractility.

Adverse effects
- *Common*: constipation, headache, ankle swelling
- *Rare*: cardiac failure, hypotension, AV node block

Contraindications
- Ventricular tachycardia (potentially lethal with verapamil)
- Heart failure/cardiogenic shock
- Hypotension
- Myocardial conduction defects (e.g. bradycardia, AV node block)

Interactions
- *Amiodarone*: concomitant use of amiodarone and verapamil increases the risk of bradycardia, AV block and myocardial depression
- ***Antihypertensives***: verapamil enhances the hypotensive effect of other antihypertensives
- ***β blockers***: if β blockers are given with or prior to verapamil there is an increased risk of AV node block which may be complete and result in asystole, heart failure and severe hypotension
- *Cyclosporin*: verapamil increases the plasma concentration of cyclosporin
- ***Digoxin***: verapamil increases the plasma concentration of digoxin

Route of administration
- Oral, IV (paroxysmal tachydysrhythmia only)

Note
- β blockers are the preferred treatment in unstable angina as they have been shown to reduce the associated risk of myocardial infarction (unlike verapamil). However, if β blockers are ineffective verapamil can be used.

Related drugs
- Diltiazem

Warfarin

Class: Oral anticoagulant (vitamin K antagonist)

Indications
- Prevention of thrombo-embolism (e.g. in atrial fibrillation, prosthetic heart valves)
- Treatment and prevention of deep vein thrombosis and pulmonary embolism
- Prevention of transient ischaemic attacks

Mechanism of action
- Vitamin K is an essential cofactor for synthesis of clotting factors II, VII, IX and X, and proteins C and S. Warfarin competitively antagonizes vitamin K and thus inhibits production of these clotting factors.
- Warfarin takes at least 48–72 hours to achieve its full anticoagulant effect (this reflects the half-life of the clotting factors).

Adverse effects
- *Common*: haemorrhage
- *Rare*: skin necrosis, liver damage, alopecia, pancreatitis, hypersensitivity, diarrhoea, nausea, vomiting

Contraindications
- Pregnancy
- Severe hypertension
- Active peptic ulcer disease
- Recent stroke
- Endocarditis

Interactions
- ***Alcohol***, *amiodarone, cimetidine, omeprazole and simvastatin*: these drugs increase the anticoagulant effect of warfarin
- ***Aspirin***: concomitant use of aspirin and warfarin results in an increased risk of haemorrhage
- *Carbamazepine, rifampicin*: these drugs decrease the anticoagulant effect of warfarin
- ***COC pill***: the COC pill decreases the anticoagulant effect of warfarin
- *Note*: Warfarin is metabolized by hepatic enzymes which can be induced or inhibited by other drugs, hence a wide range of further interactions exists

Route of administration
- Oral

Note
- Therapy should be assessed regularly by measuring INR. The target INR varies with different conditions.
- Warfarin may rarely cause fetal abnormalities if taken during pregnancy (e.g. chondrodysplasia punctata).
- In severe haemorrhage warfarin should be stopped and IV vitamin K with clotting factors II, VII, IX and X should be given. If clotting factors are unavailable, fresh frozen plasma can be used.

Related drugs
- Nicoumalone, phenindione

RESPIRATORY SYSTEM

This chapter provides an account of the management of acute
and chronic asthma and COPD. This is followed by a detailed
description of important individual drugs used in these
conditions.

ACUTE ASTHMA
- Therapy is guided by clinical state (e.g. heart rate,
respiratory rate, ability to complete sentences, blood pressure)
and peak expiratory flow rate
- Give 60% oxygen through face mask
- Give nebulized salbutamol
- Give IV hydrocortisone or oral prednisolone
- Take arterial blood gases to assess severity of the attack
- Take a chest X-ray to exclude other conditions (e.g.
pneumothorax, pneumonia)
- Check response to treatment by monitoring oxygen
saturation, measuring peak expiratory flow rate and
repeating arterial blood gases
- If the patient is deteriorating (e.g. decreasing peak
expiratory flow rate):
    - Add ipratropium bromide to the salbutamol nebulizer
    - If no improvement, consider IV aminophylline
    (contraindicated if taking oral theophylline) or IV
    salbutamol
    - If, despite this, the patient fails to improve (especially if
    PCO_2 is rising), transfer to ITU and consider mechanical
    ventilation
- If the patient is improving conduct the following until
stabilized:
    - Give oxygen and nebulized salbutamol every 4 hours
    - Give daily oral prednisolone or 6-hourly IV
    hydrocortisone
- Before discharge from hospital consider stepping up usual
treatment (see chronic asthma), educating about compliance
and checking inhaler technique

CHRONIC ASTHMA
- Start therapy at step 1 and proceed to the next step if
treatment fails to control the symptoms:
    - Step 1: β_2 agonist (e.g. salbutamol) as required
    - Step 2: inhaled β_2 agonist as required + regular sodium
    cromoglycate; or β_2 agonist as required + regular low
    dose inhaled corticosteroid (e.g. beclomethasone)
    - Step 3: inhaled β_2 agonist as required + regular high dose
    inhaled corticosteroid; or a long-acting β_2 agonist + low
    dose inhaled steroid

- Step 4: inhaled β_2 agonist as required + regular high dose inhaled corticosteroid + one or more of the following regularly:
    1 Inhaled ipratropium
    2 Oral theophylline
    3 Leukotriene antagonist
  - Step 5: add regular oral corticosteroid (prednisolone)
- Review treatment every 3–6 months

CHRONIC OBSTRUCTIVE PULMONARY DISEASE
- Advise to stop smoking
- Spirometry is useful to assess disease severity and monitor progression
- Consider a 2 week corticosteroid trial to assess if any reversible obstruction is present
- If reversible obstruction is present, the following may be given in various combinations:
    - Inhaled ipratropium
    - Bronchodilators (e.g. salbutamol)
    - Inhaled corticosteroids (e.g. beclomethasone)
    - Oral theophylline
- For acute exacerbations give appropriate antibiotics and consider hospital admission
- Consider chest physiotherapy to prevent accumulation of secretions
- Prophylactic pneumococcal and influenza vaccine can be given
- Prescribe long term oxygen therapy if indicated
- Diuretics can be used to treat any associated cor pulmonale (right-sided heart failure secondary to chronic lung disease)
- *Note*: The use of inhaled corticosteroids in COPD is a controversial issue—many believe they are of no value as COPD is a different disease process to asthma

Beclomethasone

Class: Corticosteroid

Indications
- Prophylaxis of asthma
- Inflammatory skin disorders (e.g. eczema, psoriasis)
- Prophylaxis and treatment of allergic or vasomotor rhinitis

Mechanism of action
- Beclomethasone indirectly inhibits the formation of inflammatory mediators (e.g. prostaglandins, leukotrienes) thus decreasing inflammation.

Adverse effects
- *Common*: cough, hoarse voice, candida infection in the mouth (with the inhaler)
- *Rare*: thinning of the skin, depigmentation, acne at the site of application, nose bleeds, disturbance of smell (with long term nasal spray), glaucoma

Contraindications
- Skin ointment is contraindicated in acne vulgaris, rosacea and skin infections
- Nasal spray is contraindicated in untreated nose infections

Interactions
- None

Route of administration
- Inhaler (asthma), skin ointment (skin conditions), nasal spray (rhinitis)

Note
- Using a spacer with the inhaler can prevent oral candidiasis and hoarseness. Additionally, the mouth can be rinsed out with water after using the inhaler.
- Growth should be monitored in children on long term treatment as corticosteroids may cause growth retardation.
- The issue of high dose inhaled steroids and systemic adverse effects is controversial. Some systemic absorption does occur, even with the inhaled route.

Oxygen

Class: Therapeutic gas

Indications
- Resuscitation (up to 100% oxygen)
- High concentrations (up to 60% oxygen) are used for acute hypoxic events (e.g. myocardial infarction, acute asthma, acute poisoning, pneumonia, pulmonary embolism)
- Low concentrations (up to 28% oxygen) are used in patients with respiratory disease with CO_2 retention (e.g. COPD)

Mechanism of action
- Oxygen specifically binds to haemoglobin and also dissolves in plasma. It is then transported to tissues, where it promotes aerobic respiration.

Adverse effects
- *Rare*: respiratory arrest in COPD, pulmonary oedema, retinopathy in neonates (with high concentrations)

Contraindications
- None

Interactions
- None

Route of administration
- Inhalation by nasal cannula, face mask, tent, hood, endotracheal tube

Note
- A humidifier should be used when oxygen is given in high concentrations, as it can cause throat irritation.
- Endotracheal tube is the only definite means of delivering known concentrations of oxygen.
- Different face masks deliver different concentrations of oxygen (e.g. Venturi mask delivers 24%).
- Long term home oxygen may prolong survival in those with severe COPD and coexisting cor pulmonale (at least 15 hours of oxygen should be used per day).
- Oxygen should only be prescribed for home use after thorough evaluation by respiratory physicians in hospital. Patients using oxygen should be advised of fire risks.

Salbutamol

Class: β_2 agonist

Indications
- Asthma
- COPD with reversible component
- Premature labour

Mechanism of action
- Salbutamol stimulates β_2 adrenoceptors in the airways, which generates intracellular cyclic AMP. This decreases intracellular calcium and produces bronchodilatation (as calcium is required for bronchial smooth muscle contraction).
- Salbutamol prevents degranulation of mast cells.
- When used in premature labour, salbutamol acts by inhibiting uterine smooth muscle contraction.

Adverse effects
- *Common*: tremor, tachycardia
- *Rare*: headache, palpitations, hypokalaemia, muscle cramps, insomnia (these adverse effects are dose-dependent and therefore more common with high doses)

Contraindications
- None

Interactions
- *Corticosteroids*: high doses of corticosteroids given with high doses of salbutamol increase the risk of hypokalaemia
- *Diuretics*: high doses of salbutamol increase the risk of hypokalaemia if given with loop or thiazide diuretics
- *Theophylline*: high doses of salbutamol increase the risk of hypokalaemia if given with theophylline

Route of administration
- Asthma: inhalation (aerosol, powder, nebulized solution), IM, IV, subcutaneous, oral
- COPD: inhalation
- Premature labour: IM or IV

Note
- Plasma potassium concentration needs to be monitored if salbutamol is given in severe asthma. This is due to the increased risk of hypokalaemia caused by high doses of salbutamol, hypoxia and concomitant treatment with diuretics and theophylline.
- Metered-dose inhalers are only useful in patients over 8 years of age. If younger, use a spacer or a nebulizer to administer inhaled salbutamol.

Related drugs
- Shorter-acting β_2 antagonists: bambuterol, fenoterol, reproterol, terbutaline, tulobuterol
- Longer-acting β_2 antagonists: eformoterol, salmeterol

Sodium cromoglycate

Class: Mast cell stabilizer

Indications
- Prophylaxis of asthma
- Allergic rhinitis
- Allergic conjunctivitis
- Food allergy

Mechanism of action
- Exact mechanism is not fully understood.
- Sodium cromoglycate may reduce calcium influx into mast cells, thus rendering them more stable, i.e. less likely to release inflammatory mediators. This occurs in the bronchial tree, the nose and the eyes.

Adverse effects
- *Common*: cough, throat irritation, transient bronchospasm (with inhaled route)
- *Rare*: nausea, vomiting, joint pain, rash (with oral administration), stinging of the eyes (with eye drops)

Contraindications
- None

Interactions
- None

Route of administration
- Asthma: aerosol, powder or nebulized solution
- Food allergy: oral
- Allergic rhinitis: nasal spray
- Allergic conjunctivitis: eye drops

Note
- Sodium cromoglycate is not used in acute exacerbations of asthma.
- Sodium cromoglycate is generally less effective than inhaled corticosteroids in the prophylaxis of asthma in adults. It is therefore not commonly used in adult asthma.
- Roughly one third of patients taking sodium cromoglycate, especially children, benefit from it.
- Sodium cromoglycate is useful in the prevention of asthma induced by exercise.
- If transient bronchospasm is a problem, a β_2 agonist can be inhaled a few minutes before sodium cromoglycate.
- Throat irritation can be avoided by rinsing the mouth with water after inhalation.

Related drugs
- Nedocromil sodium

Theophylline

Class: Methylxanthine

Indications
- Asthma (including acute severe asthma)
- COPD

Mechanism of action
- Bronchodilatation is thought to be achieved by a variety of mechanisms, including inhibition of the enzyme phosphodiesterase, which degrades cyclic AMP. The raised cyclic AMP levels decrease intracellular calcium, resulting in bronchodilatation.
- Theophylline also blocks adenosine receptors which results in smooth muscle relaxation in the bronchi.
- It is further believed to inhibit inflammatory cells such as mast cells.

Adverse effects
- *Common*: nausea, vomiting, headache, palpitations
- *Rare*: hypokalaemia, diarrhoea, CNS stimulation (insomnia, irritability, fine tremor), convulsions, dysrhythmias

Contraindications
- None
- Caution:
  - Cardiac disease (risk of dysrhythmias)
  - Hypertension
  - Epilepsy

Interactions
- ***Clarithromycin***: clarithromycin increases the plasma concentration of theophylline
- ***Diltiazem, verapamil***: these increase the plasma concentration of theophylline
- ***Erythromycin***: erythromycin increases the plasma concentration of theophylline
- *Note*: Theophylline is metabolized by hepatic enzymes which can be induced or inhibited by other drugs, hence a wide range of further interactions exists

Route of administration
- Oral, IV (in acute severe asthma)

Note
- Therapeutic drug monitoring is recommended.
- Oral sustained-release tablets are available, which are effective for up to 12 hours (less adverse effects).
- Theophylline can be given in combination with ethylenediamine as aminophylline. This is more readily absorbed and has fewer GI adverse effects.
- Plasma levels of theophylline should be measured if given with aminophylline due to the risk of severe adverse effects (e.g. convulsions or dysrhythmias).

Related drugs
- Aminophylline (the most widely used methylxanthine)

GASTROINTESTINAL SYSTEM

This chapter provides an account of the management of common GI conditions followed by a detailed description of important individual drugs.

PEPTIC ULCER
- Reduce exacerbating factors (e.g. smoking, obesity, alcohol, spicy foods)
- Stop NSAIDs (if appropriate)
- Give antacids for pain relief (e.g. magnesium salts, aluminium salts)
- Give an H_2 antagonist for 4–8 weeks (e.g. cimetidine)
- Endoscopy should be performed if no response to H_2 antagonist, especially if over 45 years of age (to exclude malignancy)
- If still symptomatic give a proton pump inhibitor for 4–8 weeks (e.g. omeprazole)
- Other treatment options include anticholinergics (e.g. pirenzipine), prostaglandin analogues (e.g. misoprostol), ulcer-healing agents (e.g. bismuth, sucralfate, carbenoxolone)
- If still symptomatic, treat as for *Helicobacter pylori* infection (see below)
- In resistant cases consider surgery (gastrectomy, vagotomy or pyloroplasty)

HELICOBACTER PYLORI INFECTION
- Triple therapy for 2 weeks (many combinations exist, three of which are shown here):
    1 Omeprazole, metronidazole and amoxycillin
    2 Omeprazole, clarithromycin and amoxycillin
    3 Lansoprazole, clarithromycin and metronidazole

CONSTIPATION
- Treat any underlying cause
- Recommend high fibre diet with adequate fluid intake
- If the above fails, consider any one of the following laxatives:
    - Bulking agents (e.g. bran)
    - Stool softeners (e.g. arachis oil)
    - Stimulant laxatives (e.g. senna)
    - Osmotic laxatives (e.g. lactulose)

DIARRHOEA
- Remember that most cases of diarrhoea are self-limiting
- Aim of treatment is to replace fluid and electrolyte loss by oral rehydration therapy (IV in nausea and vomiting)

- Treat any underlying cause
- The following can be given for symptomatic relief, if the cause is unknown:
  - Loperamide
  - Codeine phosphate
  - Diphenoxylate
- Send a stool sample for microbiology if infection is suspected
- Investigate with sigmoidoscopy or colonoscopy if diarrhoea lasts longer than 6 weeks

CROHN'S DISEASE
- Only treat flare-ups
- For minor flare-ups give an oral corticosteroid (e.g. prednisolone)
- For major flare-ups give IV corticosteroids (e.g. prednisolone), IV fluids and consider elemental diet by nasogastric tube (liquid preparation of amino acids, fat and carbohydrates)
- 5-ASA agents (e.g. sulphasalazine) may be beneficial in small bowel Crohn's disease
- In patients with chronic Crohn's disease consider azathioprine and corticosteroids to maintain remission

ULCERATIVE COLITIS
- Give a 5-ASA preparation as maintenance therapy (e.g. sulphasalazine)
- For minor flare-ups give rectal corticosteroids (e.g. prednisolone) and rectal 5-ASA
- For severe flare-ups give oral or IV corticosteroids (e.g. prednisolone), 5-ASA and IV fluids
- If still symptomatic consider azathioprine

Antacids

(Aluminium salts, magnesium salts, sodium bicarbonate)

Indications
- Symptomatic relief of:
  - Non-ulcer dyspepsia (e.g. due to indigestion, gastric cancer)
  - Gastric or duodenal ulcer
  - Gastro-oesophageal reflux disease
- Acidosis (sodium bicarbonate is used)

Mechanism of action
- Antacids are weak alkalis, which neutralize the acid in the stomach.
- Some antacids are combined with alginates to further suppress acid reflux (alginates protect the oesophagus by forming a 'raft', which decreases acid regurgitation).

Adverse effects
- *Common*: constipation (aluminium salts), diarrhoea (magnesium salts), belching (sodium bicarbonate)
- *Rare*: metabolic alkalosis, increased risk of developing phosphate-containing renal stones, worsened or precipitated heart failure or hypertension (all with sodium bicarbonate)

Contraindications
- Hypophosphataemia (aluminium and magnesium salts)
- Caution:
  - Salt restriction diet (sodium bicarbonate)
  - Renal impairment (magnesium salts)

Interactions
- *ACE inhibitors, antibacterials, digoxin, iron*: antacids decrease the absorption of these drugs
- *Lithium*: sodium bicarbonate increases the excretion of lithium, thus decreasing its plasma concentration

Route of administration
- Oral

Note
- Most antacids are not absorbed from the GI tract and therefore rarely cause systemic adverse effects.

Cimetidine

Class: Histamine (H_2) antagonist

Indications
- Gastric and duodenal ulcers
- Gastro-oesophageal reflux disease

Mechanism of action
- Cimetidine decreases gastric acid production. It does so by acting as a competitive antagonist at histamine (H_2) receptors on parietal cells in the stomach.
- Cimetidine also increases prolactin levels and has anti-androgenic properties. This may lead to adverse effects.

Adverse effects
- *Rare*: diarrhoea, dizziness, impotence, galactorrhoea, amenorrhoea, gynaecomastia, testicular atrophy, cardiac dysrhythmias (if given IV), rash

Contraindications
- None

Interactions
- *Anticonvulsants (carbamazepine, phenytoin, sodium valproate)*: cimetidine increases the plasma concentration of these drugs by inhibiting their metabolism
- *Cyclosporin*: cimetidine increases the plasma concentration of cyclosporin, resulting in serious adverse effects
- *Theophylline*: cimetidine increases the plasma concentration of theophylline by inhibiting its metabolism
- *Warfarin*: cimetidine increases the anticoagulant effect of warfarin by inhibiting its metabolism
- *Note*: Cimetidine inhibits hepatic drug metabolizing enzymes, hence a wide range of further interactions exists

Route of administration
- Oral, IM, IV

Note
- Treatment should last for 4–8 weeks, after which most ulcers should have healed. If not, *Helicobacter pylori* testing and eradication should be considered.
- Gastric cancer must be excluded before prescribing cimetidine to elderly and middle-aged patients as cimetidine may mask the symptoms and thus delay diagnosis.
- Ranitidine is a preferred alternative to cimetidine because it has fewer adverse effects and fewer drug interactions. It can be safely prescribed to young males and the elderly.

Related drugs
- Famotidine, nizatidine, ranitidine (unlike cimetidine, these are not hepatic enzyme inhibitors)

Ferrous sulphate

Class: Iron salt

Indications
- Iron-deficiency anaemia

Mechanism of action
- Ferrous sulphate replenishes iron stores.

Adverse effects
- *Common*: nausea, epigastric pain, constipation or diarrhoea, darkening of faeces (often confused with melaena)

Contraindications
- None
- Caution:
  - Pregnancy

Interactions
- *Tetracycline*: absorption of ferrous sulphate is decreased by tetracycline

Route of administration
- Oral

Note
- The cause of iron-deficiency anaemia should be sought prior to administration of ferrous sulphate.
- Haemoglobin concentration increases by roughly 2 g/dL every 3 weeks with treatment.
- Iron deficiency causes hypochromic microcytic anaemia with low serum ferritin levels and increased total iron binding capacity (TIBC).
- In order to replenish iron stores, treatment with oral ferrous sulphate is continued for 3–6 months after haemoglobin levels have reached the normal range.
- Patients unable to tolerate oral iron (e.g. because of severe adverse effects) should be given iron sorbitol by deep IM injection.
- Absorption of ferrous sulphate can be improved by combining it with vitamin C.
- Potentially fatal iron poisoning (nausea, vomiting, bloody diarrhoea, haematemesis, abdominal pain, hypotension and coma) is commonest in children. Gastric lavage should be performed at once and desferrioxamine (which chelates iron) should be administered.

Related drugs
- Ferrous fumarate, ferrous gluconate

Folic acid

Class: Vitamin supplement

Indications
- Prevention of neural tube defects in pregnancy
- Folate-deficient megaloblastic anaemia
- End-stage renal failure
- Chronic haemolytic states
- Prevention of folate deficiency in patients taking anticonvulsants

Mechanism of action
- Folic acid has a role in cell metabolism because of its ability to transfer single carbon atom-containing groups. This is important in the synthesis of purines and pyrimidines and therefore in the synthesis of DNA.

Adverse effects
- None

Contraindications
- Folic acid alone should not be given to patients with anaemia secondary to vitamin B_{12} deficiency as this may precipitate subacute combined degeneration of the spinal cord. In this case it should be administered in conjunction with vitamin B_{12}.

Interactions
- No serious interactions

Route of administration
- Oral

Note
- The cause of folate deficiency should be ascertained and corrected prior to folate therapy.
- Folate is absorbed in the proximal jejunum. Folate deficiency is therefore a leading finding in coeliac disease.
- In order to prevent neural tube defects, women should be given daily folic acid supplements prior to conception and also until the 12th week of pregnancy.

Hydroxocobalamin

Class: Vitamin B_{12}

Indications
- Pernicious anaemia
- Other vitamin B_{12}-deficiency states (e.g. following gastrectomy or total ileal resection)
- Schilling test

Mechanism of action
- Hydroxocobalamin is needed for synthesis of purines and pyrimidines and their subsequent incorporation into DNA.

Adverse effects
- *Rare*: anaphylaxis, nausea, dizziness, pruritus, fever

Contraindications
- None

Interactions
- None

Route of administration
- IM

Note
- Hydroxocobalamin has replaced cyanocobalamin as therapeutic vitamin B_{12} because it is retained in the body for a longer period.
- Vitamin B_{12} is absorbed in the terminal ileum.
- Schilling test is employed in the diagnosis of pernicious anaemia.
- Hydroxocobalamin injections are given on alternate days for the first few weeks and once every 3 months thereafter.

Lactulose

Class: Osmotic laxative

Indications
- Constipation
- Hepatic encephalopathy

Mechanism of action
- Lactulose is a disaccharide consisting of fructose and galactose.
- Lactulose stimulates peristalsis by increasing the volume of intestinal contents. It cannot be metabolized by human disaccharidases, but is hydrolysed to glucose and galactose by bacteria in the colon. These draw water by osmosis into the intestinal lumen.
- Lactulose also decreases the pH of the gut contents, thus reducing the activity of ammonia-producing organisms, hence its use in hepatic encephalopathy (ammonia is thought to cross the blood–brain barrier and act as a false neurotransmitter, thus causing the symptoms of hepatic encephalopathy).

Adverse effects
- *Common*: flatulence, abdominal cramps, belching, diarrhoea
- *Rare*: abdominal distension

Contraindications
- Intestinal obstruction
- Galactosaemia

Interactions
- None (as it is not absorbed)

Route of administration
- Oral

Note
- Lactulose needs about 48 hours to have an effect.
- It can be given to prevent constipation in opiate therapy.

Loperamide

Class: Opiate antimotility drug

Indications
- Supplement to rehydration in acute diarrhoea (patients over 4 years of age only)
- Chronic diarrhoea (adults only)

Mechanism of action
- Loperamide acts on opioid μ receptors in the myenteric plexus of the gut wall. This inhibits acetylcholine release from the myenteric plexus and hence inhibits peristalsis.

Adverse effects
- *Rare*: constipation, abdominal pain, bloating, rash, paralytic ileus

Contraindications
- Active ulcerative colitis
- Antibiotic-associated colitis
- Dysentery

Interactions
- None

Route of administration
- Oral

Note
- Loperamide should not be used for long periods. Further investigation into the cause of diarrhoea should be considered if no improvement is evident after 2 days of treatment.
- Unlike other opioids, loperamide does not easily penetrate the blood–brain barrier, which makes it unlikely to cause central effects and dependence.

Related drugs
- Codeine phosphate, cophenotrope, morphine

Metoclopramide

Class: Dopamine (D_2) antagonist

Indications
  • Nausea and vomiting (due to opioids, chemotherapy, radiotherapy, migraine or postoperatively)
  • Gastro-oesophageal reflux

Mechanism of action
  • Metoclopramide has several actions, all of which contribute to its anti-emetic effect:
    1 It blocks dopamine (D_2) receptors in the chemoreceptor trigger zone in the brain stem.
    2 It increases the rate of gastric and duodenal emptying by causing relaxation of the pyloric sphincter. It also increases lower oesophageal sphincter tone.

Adverse effects
  • *Common*: acute dystonic reactions (e.g. oculogyric crisis) especially in children and young adults
  • *Rare*: tardive dyskinesia, depression, galactorrhoea, cardiac conduction abnormalities, drowsiness, restlessness, diarrhoea

Contraindications
  • Parkinsonism
  • the first 3–4 days following gastrointestinal surgery
  • Intestinal obstruction

Interactions
  • *Lithium*: metoclopramide increases the risk of extrapyramidal adverse effects
  • *NSAIDs*: metoclopramide increases the absorption of NSAIDs, thus enhancing their effects

Route of administration
  • Oral, IM, IV

Note
  • Nausea and vomiting in migraine can cause gastric stasis which reduces the absorption rate of aspirin and paracetamol. In order to accelerate their absorption, aspirin and paracetamol can be combined with metoclopramide.
  • Acute dystonic reactions are especially common in young females taking metoclopramide. These can be treated with a muscarinic antagonist (e.g. benztropine).
  • Domperidone has similar pharmacological actions, but is less likely to cause CNS effects due to its poor transport across the blood–brain barrier.

Related drugs
  • Domperidone

Omeprazole

Class: Proton-pump inhibitor

Indications
- Gastro-oesophageal reflux/oesophagitis
- Gastric or duodenal ulcer
- Part of *Helicobacter pylori* eradication therapy
- Zollinger–Ellison syndrome

Mechanism of action
- Omeprazole causes dose-dependent irreversible inhibition of gastric acid production by inhibiting the H^+/K^+ ATPase ('proton pump') in gastric parietal cells. Acid secretion is thus inhibited by $> 90\%$.
- Omeprazole is activated at low pH.

Adverse effects
- *Common*: headache, diarrhoea
- *Rare*: constipation, nausea, vomiting, rash

Contraindications
- None
- Caution:
  - Liver disease
  - Pregnancy
  - Breast feeding

Interactions
- **Phenytoin**: omeprazole increases the plasma concentration of phenytoin
- **Warfarin**: omeprazole increases the plasma concentration of warfarin
- *Note*: Omeprazole inhibits hepatic drug-metabolizing enzymes, hence a wide range of further interactions exists

Route of administration
- Oral

Note
- Achlorhydria is linked with gastric cancer and for this reason some physicians are concerned about long term therapy with proton-pump inhibitors.
- Omeprazole may mask gastric cancer. It is therefore important to exclude malignancy before treatment.
- Omeprazole is more efficient at reducing gastric acidity and has a longer duration of action than histamine (H_2) antagonists.

Related drugs
- Lansoprazole, pantoprazole, rabeprazole

Ondansetron

Class: Serotonin (5-HT$_3$) antagonist

Indications
- Treatment and prophylaxis of nausea and vomiting (in chemotherapy, radiotherapy and postoperatively)

Mechanism of action
- Exact mechanism is not fully understood.
- Ondansetron selectively blocks excitatory serotonin receptors in the chemoreceptor trigger zone of the brain and in the GI tract.

Adverse effects
- *Common*: headache, constipation
- *Rare*: flushing, sedation, abdominal discomfort

Contraindications
- None
- Caution:
  - Pregnancy
  - Breast feeding
  - Hepatic impairment

Interactions
- None

Route of administration
- Oral, IM, IV, rectal

Note
- Ondansetron can be used in conjunction with corticosteroids for chemotherapy-induced nausea and vomiting.

Related drugs
- Granisetron, tropisetron

Pancreatin

Class: Enzyme-containing pancreas extract

Indications
- Reduced or absent pancreatic exocrine secretions (e.g. in cystic fibrosis, chronic pancreatitis, following pancreatectomy)

Mechanism of action
- Pancreatin contains trypsin and chymotrypsin (for breakdown of proteins), amylase (for breakdown of starch) and lipase (for breakdown of fats).
- These enzymes are essential for an efficient digestive process.

Adverse effects
- *Rare*: nausea, vomiting, diarrhoea, abdominal discomfort, hypersensitivity, perianal irritation (with excessive doses)

Contraindications
- None

Interactions
- No serious interactions

Route of administration
- Oral

Note
- Pancreatin should be taken with food. Additionally, histamine (H_2) receptor antagonists (e.g. ranitidine) or antacids can be given in conjunction with pancreatin to prevent destruction of the pancreatic enzymes by gastric acid.
- Excessive heat inactivates the enzymes contained in pancreatin. It should not be mixed with hot foods or liquids.
- Enteric-coated preparations carry more of the enzymes to the duodenum. This makes pancreatin therapy more efficient.

Senna

Class: Stimulant laxative

Indications
- Constipation

Mechanism of action
- Senna is hydrolysed by bacteria in the colon to produce irritant anthracene glycoside derivatives. These stimulate the myenteric (Auerbach's) plexus in the gut wall to increase peristalsis.

Adverse effects
- *Common*: abdominal cramps, diarrhoea
- *Rare*: hypokalaemia, colonic atony (with prolonged use)

Contraindications
- Intestinal obstruction

Interactions
- None

Route of administration
- Oral

Note
- Senna acts in 8–12 hours.
- Regular use of senna can lead to tolerance and should therefore be used for short periods only.
- Patients taking senna should be warned about the dangers of continuous purgation (e.g. hypokalaemia, atonic colon) and the need for regular bowel habits.
- A high fibre intake (e.g. fruit, vegetable, whole wheat) should be encouraged.

Related drugs
- Bisacodyl, docusate sodium, glycerol, oxyphenisatin, sodium picosulphate

Sulphasalazine

Class: Aminosalicylate

Indications
- Ulcerative colitis (treatment and maintenance of remission)
- Active Crohn's disease
- Rheumatoid arthritis

Mechanism of action
- Sulphasalazine is split into 5-aminosalicylic acid (5-ASA) and sulphapyridine (a sulphonamide) by colonic flora. The function of sulphapyridine is to carry 5-ASA to the gut. 5-ASA is an active anti-inflammatory agent whose mechanism of action in the large bowel is not yet clear.
- In rheumatoid arthritis, it is the sulphapyridine component which acts as a disease-modifying antirheumatic drug.

Adverse effects
- *Common*: nausea, abdominal discomfort, anorexia
- *Rare*: blood dyscrasias, low sperm count, tinnitus, acute pancreatitis, hepatitis, hypersensitivity

Contraindications
- Salicylate hypersensitivity
- Renal impairment
- Children under the age of 2 years

Interactions
- No serious interactions

Route of administration
- Oral, rectal

Note
- As high doses of sulphasalazine are usually required, adverse effects can be minimized by increasing the dose slowly and using enteric-coated tablets.
- The risk of GI adverse effects can be reduced by maintaining an adequate fluid intake.
- Patients should be advised to report unexplained bleeding, bruising or sore throat. If these symptoms occur, a blood count should be performed to exclude any blood dyscrasias.
- Newer aminosalicylates, such as mesalazine or olsalazine, have fewer adverse effects. This is because they lack the sulphonamide component, which is responsible for most of the adverse effects.

Related drugs
- Mesalazine, olsalazine

CENTRAL NERVOUS SYSTEM

This chapter provides an account of the management of common neurological conditions followed by a description of important drugs used in psychiatry and neurology.

MIGRAINE
Acute attacks
- Give paracetamol or soluble aspirin
- Metoclopramide can be given for associated nausea and vomiting (and also to increase the rate of absorption of aspirin and paracetamol)
- Consider sumatriptan nasal spray or oral rizatriptan if the above fails

Prophylaxis
- Avoid precipitating factors (mainly emotional factors, but also chocolate, cheese, alcohol)
- Prophylaxis is given to patients who experience more than one severe migraine attack per month
- Give propranolol or a tricyclic antidepressant (e.g. amitriptyline)
- Consider a serotonin antagonist (e.g. pizotifen)

DEPRESSION
- Treat only if the patient is clinically depressed
- First line therapy: TCA (e.g. amitriptyline) or a SSRI (e.g. fluoxetine)
- If still symptomatic consider changing to a MAOI (e.g. phenelzine)
- If still symptomatic consider combination therapy of MAOI + TCA *or* SSRI + TCA
- Improvement is not usually seen until 4–6 weeks after starting treatment
- Continue therapy for at least 6 months and then review
- For rapid effect and for patients not responding to antidepressants consider electroconvulsive therapy (ECT)
- Psychotherapy and counselling may be of benefit to some patients

EPILEPSY
Partial seizures
- 1st line therapy: give carbamazepine or sodium valproate
- 2nd line therapy: give lamotrigine or phenytoin or topiramate
- Adjunctive therapy: gabapentin

Generalized seizures
- Absence seizures: give sodium valproate or ethosuximide

- Tonic/clonic seizures: give carbamazepine or sodium valproate or phenytoin
- Myoclonic and atonic seizures: give sodium valproate or clonazepam

Status epilepticus
- Give oxygen through face mask
- Give IV diazepam (rectal if IV access not possible)
- If no response repeat IV diazepam
- Give 50 mL of 50% dextrose IV if blood glucose is low
- If still fitting add IV fosphenytoin (enters the brain more rapidly than phenytoin)
- If still fitting after maximum dose of diazepam and phenytoin consider phenobarbitone, get expert help and consider mechanical ventilation under anaesthesia

IDIOPATHIC PARKINSON'S DISEASE
Supportive treatment
- Physiotherapy may be helpful in maintaining joint and muscle mobility and ensuring independence

Pharmacological treatment
- Anti-Parkinsonian drugs improve quality of life by alleviating symptoms, but they do not prevent progression of the disease
- Treatment of choice: levodopa with a peripheral decarboxylase inhibitor (e.g. benserazide)
- Dopamine agonists (e.g. ropinirole, bromocriptine, lysuride) are reserved for cases where levodopa is no longer effective or no longer tolerated
- Selegiline (MAO type B inhibitor) can be used early in the disease process or combined with levodopa to reduce 'end of dose deterioration'
- Anticholinergics (e.g. benzhexol) are used in drug-induced Parkinsonism and if tremor is a prominent symptom
- Apomorphine (dopamine agonist) can be given subcutaneously in end-stage disease
- Adjuvant treatment: entacapone (MAOI), amantadine

Drug classes

BENZODIAZEPINES
Types of Benzodiazepines
1 Short-acting: midazolam
2 Intermediate-acting: temazepam
3 Long-acting: diazepam, clonazepam

Indications
- Benzodiazepines are mainly used according to their duration of action:

- Anxiety (diazepam)
- Insomnia (temazepam)
- Convulsions (diazepam in status epilepticus, clonazepam for prophylaxis)
- Sedation for medical procedures (midazolam)
- Alcohol withdrawal (diazepam)

Mechanism of action
- BDZs potentiate the inhibitory actions of GABA by binding to GABA receptors in the CNS.

Adverse effects
- Psychological and physical dependence (especially with short-acting BDZs)
- Respiratory depression

NEUROLEPTICS
Types of neuroleptics
1 Typical
   - Phenothiazines: chlorpromazine
   - Butyrophenones: haloperidol
   - Thioxanthines: flupenthixol
2 Atypical
   - Clozapine, olanzapine, risperidone

Indications
- Psychosis
- In schizophrenia:
   - Typicals are effective for positive symptoms
   - Atypicals are effective for both negative and positive symptoms

Mechanism of action
- All neuroleptics block D_2 receptors in the brain. This is thought to be responsible for the antipsychotic effect.

Adverse effects
- *Psychological*: depression
- *Neurological*: Parkinsonism, akathisia, dystonia, tardive dyskinesia (these are due to blockade of D_1 receptors)
- *Autonomic*:
   - Dry mouth, blurred vision (these are due to blockade of muscarinic receptors)
   - Postural hypotension (this is due to blockade of α_1 adrenoceptors)
- *Histamine (H_1) receptor blockade*: sedation
- *Dopamine receptor blockade*: hyperprolactinaemia and its effects (e.g. impotence, amenorrhoea)
- A rare but serious adverse effect is neuroleptic malignant syndrome
- Clozapine is associated with a risk of agranulocytosis and patients must therefore be monitored with regular blood counts
- Atypicals may be better tolerated than typical neuroleptics

Amitriptyline

Class: Tricyclic antidepressant (TCA)

Indications
- Depression
- Neuralgia
- Nocturnal enuresis in children

Mechanism of action
- Amitriptyline increases serotonin and norepinephrine transmission in the CNS. It does so by inhibiting re-uptake of these neurotransmitters from the synaptic cleft.
- Amitriptyline also blocks histamine (H_1), muscarinic and α receptors, which can result in a wide range of adverse effects.

Adverse effects
- *Common*: sedation, dry mouth, blurred vision, postural hypotension, constipation
- *Rare*: convulsions, dysrhythmias, heart block, weight gain, difficulty in passing urine, precipitation of glaucoma

Contraindications
- Epilepsy
- Recent myocardial infarction
- Severe coronary heart disease
- Dysrhythmias (especially heart block)
- Mania and other severe psychiatric conditions

Interactions
- *Anti-arrhythmics*: amitriptyline increases the risk of ventricular dysrhythmias with anti-arrhythmics
- *Anticonvulsants*: amitriptyline antagonizes the anticonvulsant effect
- *MAOIs*: danger of potentially fatal hyperthermia syndrome
- *Neuroleptics*: increased risk of ventricular dysrhythmias if neuroleptics are given with TCAs

Route of administration
- Depression: oral, IV, IM
- Neuralgia and nocturnal enuresis: oral

Note
- SSRIs are sometimes preferred to TCAs as they are safer in overdose and may have less severe adverse effects.
- Amitriptyline must be taken regularly for 3–4 weeks before any improvement is likely.
- Treatment should be continued for at least 6 months to prevent recurrence of depression, even if the patient has recovered.
- Sedative properties of amitriptyline are useful in depression associated with insomnia.

Related drugs
- Clomipramine, dothiepin, trimipramine (these have sedative properties)
- Imipramine, lofepramine, nortriptyline (these have less sedative properties)

Bromocriptine

Class: Dopamine agonist

Indications
- Idiopathic Parkinson's disease
- Hyperprolactinaemia
- Acromegaly
- Cyclical benign breast disease
- Prevention and suppression of lactation

Mechanism of action
- Bromocriptine stimulates dopamine receptors in the CNS. These are normally stimulated by dopamine, which is deficient in Parkinson's disease.
- Bromocriptine is useful in hyperprolactinaemia as it inhibits the release of prolactin from the anterior pituitary gland. This inhibits lactation.
- Bromocriptine inhibits the release of growth hormone in acromegaly (in unaffected individuals growth hormone levels are raised by bromocriptine).

Adverse effects
- *Common*: nausea, vomiting, constipation, postural hypotension
- *Rare*: confusion, drowsiness, dyskinesia

Contraindications
- Hypersensitivity
- Drug-induced Parkinsonism

Interactions
- *Erythromycin*: erythromycin increases the plasma concentration of bromocriptine, thus increasing the risk of dose-dependent adverse effects
- *Sympathomimetics (epinephrine, isoprenalin, dobutamine, dopamine)*: sympathomimetics increase the risk of adverse effects of bromocriptine

Route of administration
- Oral

Note
- Nausea and vomiting can be decreased by increasing the dose of bromocriptine slowly and taking it with meals.
- High doses of bromocriptine are normally used in the treatment of acromegaly and Parkinson's disease. This entails a greater occurrence of adverse effects.
- Domperidone can be used to reduce the systemic adverse effects of bromocriptine. It does not reduce central adverse effects as it does not cross the blood–brain barrier.
- Bromocriptine can decrease the size of prolactinoma tumours as well as reduce the prolactin plasma concentration.

Carbamazepine

Class: Anticonvulsant

Indications
- Generalized tonic-clonic seizures
- Partial seizures
- Trigeminal neuralgia and other chronic neurogenic pain
- Prophylaxis of bipolar disorder

Mechanism of action
- Carbamazepine is thought to:

  1 Enhance GABA-mediated inhibitory transmission in the CNS.

  2 Decrease electrical excitability of cell membranes by blocking sodium channels.

Adverse effects
- *Common*: drowsiness, ataxia, blurred vision, confusion
- *Rare*: agranulocytosis, thrombocytopenia, hepatic failure, acute renal failure, rash, cardiac conduction abnormalities

Contraindications
- Bone marrow depression
- AV node conduction abnormalities (unless pacemaker *in situ*)
- Porphyria

Interactions
- **Cimetidine, erythromycin**: these drugs increase the plasma concentration of carbamazepine by inhibiting its metabolism
- *Corticosteroids, cyclosporin, phenytoin*: the effect of these drugs is reduced by carbamazepine
- *Diltiazem, isoniazid, verapamil*: these drugs increase the plasma concentration of carbamazepine
- **Oral contraceptive pill**: carbamazepine reduces the effect of oral contraceptives
- **Warfarin**: carbamazepine reduces the effect of warfarin
- *Note*: Carbamazepine induces hepatic drug-metabolizing enzymes, hence a wide range of further interactions exists

Route of administration
- Oral, rectal (for epilepsy, if oral route not possible)

Note
- It is important to start therapy with a low dose in order to minimize adverse effects. The dose is then increased in small increments every 2 weeks until symptoms are controlled.
- Carbamazepine can induce its own metabolism.
- Therapeutic drug monitoring is recommended.
- It is recommended to monitor blood count, hepatic function and renal function whilst on carbamazepine therapy.
- Carbamazepine is teratogenic and may cause neural tube defects in the fetus.

Chlorpromazine

Class: Phenothiazine

Indications
- Psychotic disorders (e.g. schizophrenia, mania)
- Labyrinthine disturbances and vertigo
- Nausea and vomiting
- Chronic hiccups

Mechanism of action
- Chlorpromazine has many pharmacological actions. Its use in psychotic disorders is thought to be due to blockade of dopamine receptors in the CNS (especially in the mesocortical and mesolimbic area).
- The anti-emetic effect is due to blockade of dopamine receptors in the chemoreceptor trigger zone in the brain.
- Blockade of muscarinic, histamine (H_1), serotonin and α receptors might contribute to the therapeutic action of chlorpromazine (but blockade also causes adverse effects).

Adverse effects
- *Common*: sedation, postural hypotension, increased prolactin levels (leading to subfertility, impotence, menstrual disturbances and galactorrhoea), extrapyramidal adverse effects (acute dystonia, akathisia, Parkinsonism, tardive dyskinesia with long term use), anticholinergic effects (e.g. dry mouth, blurred vision, constipation)
- *Rare*: neuroleptic malignant syndrome (hyperthermia, muscle rigidity, autonomic nervous system dysfunction), agranulocytosis, skin rash, jaundice

Contraindications
- Coma
- Bone marrow suppression
- Phaeochromocytoma

Interactions
- *ACE inhibitors:* these can cause severe postural hypotension if given with chlorpromazine

Route of administration
- Oral, rectal, IM

Note
- Compliance may be a problem in psychotic disorders. In this case slow-release preparations of other neuroleptics (e.g. haloperidol decanoate) can be given IM every few weeks.
- Extrapyramidal adverse effects are thought to be due to the blockade of dopamine receptors in the CNS.
- Chlorpromazine can be used in conjunction with an anticholinergic drug (e.g. procyclidine) to prevent short term extrapyramidal adverse effects. This, however, cannot prevent tardive dyskinesia.

Related drugs
- Fluphenazine, pipothiazine, prochlorperazine, thioridazine, trifluoperazine

Diazepam

Class: Benzodiazepine

Indications
- Anxiety
- Status epilepticus
- Febrile convulsions
- Muscle spasm (e.g. spasticity)

Mechanism of action
- Diazepam binds to GABA receptors in the CNS and thereby facilitates GABA inhibitory neurotransmission by opening chloride channels. It is thought that this action produces the anxiolytic, anticonvulsant and sedative effects.

Adverse effects
- *Common*: daytime drowsiness, confusion in the elderly
- *Rare*: headache, blurred vision, confusion, rash, thrombophlebitis (with IV injection), apnoea

Contraindications
- Respiratory depression
- Severe hepatic impairment
- Pregnancy
- Breast feeding

Interactions
- *Cimetidine*: cimetidine inhibits the metabolism of diazepam, thus increasing the risk of adverse effects of diazepam
- *Isoniazid*: isoniazid inhibits the metabolism of diazepam
- *Rifampicin*: rifampicin increases the metabolism of diazepam
- *Sedatives*: any other sedative may enhance the sedative effect of diazepam

Route of administration
- Oral, rectal (if oral route inappropriate), IM or IV (status epilepticus, acute severe anxiety)

Note
- If used for more than several weeks, diazepam can lead to tolerance and psychological/physical dependence. Therefore treatment should not exceed 2 weeks at a time.
- Abrupt withdrawal can cause anxiety, tremor, seizures and rebound sleeplessness.
- Diazepam is metabolized by the liver to active metabolites, which have very long half-lives (e.g. *N*-desmethyl diazepam has a half-life of up to 200 hours). Accumulation of active metabolites can, therefore, easily occur.
- Flumazenil is a specific benzodiazepine antagonist which can be given in diazepam overdose, but may precipitate a withdrawal syndrome.

Related drugs
- Alprazolam, bromazepam, clobazam, clonazepam, lorazepam, midazolam, nitrazepam, oxazepam

Fluoxetine

Class: Selective serotonin re-uptake inhibitor (SSRI)

Indications
- Depression
- Obsessive–compulsive disorder
- Bulimia nervosa

Mechanism of action
- Fluoxetine increases serotonin levels in the CNS by inhibiting its re-uptake from the synaptic cleft.

Adverse effects
- *Common*: headache, insomnia, nausea, diarrhoea, anxiety, sexual dysfunction
- *Rare*: anaphylaxis, drowsiness

Contraindications
- Mania

Interactions
- *Carbamazepine*: fluoxetine increases the plasma concentration of carbamazepine
- *Dopaminergics*: fluoxetine causes hypertension and CNS excitation with dopaminergics
- *Haloperidol*: fluoxetine increases the levels of haloperidol
- *Lithium*: fluoxetine increases the risk of lithium toxicity
- *MAOIs*: MAOIs enhance the CNS effects of fluoxetine (risk of hyperthermia syndrome)
- *Phenytoin*: fluoxetine increases the plasma concentration of phenytoin

Route of administration
- Oral

Note
- SSRIs are preferred to tricyclic antidepressants because they are safer in overdose. They are relatively free of anticholinergic adverse effects such as blurred vision, dry mouth and difficult micturition. They are also less sedating than tricyclic antidepressants.
- Fluoxetine should not be started until 14 days after stopping a MAOI.

Related drugs
- Citalopram, fluvoxamine, paroxetine, sertraline

Haloperidol

Class: Butyrophenone dopamine (D_2) antagonist

Indications
- Schizophrenia and other psychotic disorders
- Motor tics

Mechanism of action
- Haloperidol blocks postsynaptic dopamine (D_2) receptors in the limbic, striatal and cortical brain regions.
- It also blocks dopamine (D_1) receptors, but to a much lesser extent.

Adverse effects
- *Common*: Parkinsonism, acute dystonia, akathisia, drowsiness, postural hypotension
- *Rare*: weight loss, tardive dyskinesia, convulsions, neuroleptic malignant syndrome

Contraindications
- Coma
- Bone marrow depression

Interactions
- *Amiodarone*: haloperidol increases the risk of ventricular dysrhythmias with amiodarone
- *Carbamazepine*: carbamazepine decreases the plasma concentration of haloperidol by accelerating its metabolism
- *Fluoxetine*: fluoxetine increases the plasma concentration of haloperidol

Route of administration
- Oral, IM

Note
- Haloperidol requires several weeks before it starts to control the symptoms of schizophrenia.
- Extrapyramidal symptoms (e.g. Parkinsonism, akathisia) can be ameliorated by muscarinic antagonists (e.g. procyclidine) or by dose reduction.
- In order to avoid first-pass metabolism and improve compliance, haloperidol can be given every 1–4 weeks as a long-acting, deep depot IM injection (haloperidol decanoate).
- Haloperidol (also chlorpromazine and flupenthixol) can cause the potentially fatal neuroleptic malignant syndrome (hyperpyrexia, confusion, increased muscle tone and autonomic dysfunction). There is no effective treatment for this apart from immediate discontinuation of the drug.

Related drugs
- Benperidol, droperidol

Hyoscine

Class: Muscarinic antagonist

Indications
- Prophylaxis of motion sickness
- Intestinal spasm in irritable bowel syndrome
- Premedication (in anaesthesia)
- Eye examination (to dilate pupils)

Mechanism of action
- Hyoscine competes with acetylcholine for muscarinic receptors. This results in:
    1 Smooth muscle relaxation in bowel and the bladder
    2 Reduced secretions from bronchial and sweat glands
    3 Pupillary dilatation
    4 Bronchodilatation
    5 Increase in heart rate

Adverse effects
- *Common*: sedation, dry mouth, blurred vision
- *Rare*: constipation, difficulty with micturition, confusion, restlessness

Contraindications
- Prostatic enlargement
- Closed-angle glaucoma
- Myasthenia gravis
- Paralytic ileus
- Pyloric stenosis

Interactions
- *Alcohol*: alcohol enhances the sedative effect of hyoscine

Route of administration
- IV, IM, oral, skin patch, eye drops, subcutaneous

Note
- Muscarinic adverse effects of hyoscine can be counteracted by anticholinesterase drugs (e.g. neostigmine).

Related drugs
- Atropine (less sedating than hyoscine)

Levodopa (L-dopa)

Class: Dopamine precursor

Indications
- Idiopathic Parkinson's disease

Mechanism of action
- Levodopa crosses the blood–brain barrier and is then converted to dopamine by the enzyme dopa decarboxylase. This action replaces dopamine which is deficient in the basal ganglia in Parkinson's disease. Dopamine itself is not used, as it cannot cross the blood–brain barrier.

Adverse effects
- *Common*:
  - Systemic adverse effects—nausea, vomiting, abdominal pain, anorexia, postural hypotension, dysrhythmias, dizziness, discoloration of urine and other body fluids (all these adverse effects are reduced by adding a decarboxylase inhibitor such as benserazide or carbidopa)
  - CNS adverse effects—abnormal involuntary movements, 'on–off effect' (rigidity alternating with excessive movements)
- *Rare*: psychiatric symptoms (e.g. confusion, hallucinations, depression)

Contraindications
- Closed-angle glaucoma
- Drug-induced Parkinsonism

Interactions
- *Anaesthetics*: concomitant use of levodopa and volatile liquid anaesthetics increases the risk of dysrhythmias
- *MAOIs*: risk of hypertensive crisis if levodopa is given with MAOIs (withdraw MAOIs 2 weeks before giving levodopa)
- *Neuroleptics*: neuroleptics reduce the effects of levodopa by blocking dopamine receptors

Route of administration
- Oral

Note
- Only 1% of levodopa reaches the brain as it is peripherally converted to dopamine by dopa decarboxylase. Combining levodopa with a decarboxylase inhibitor such as benserazide or carbidopa can prevent this. Thus more dopamine reaches the brain and a reduction in systemic adverse effects is achieved.
- The efficacy of levodopa decreases with long term use. This is known as 'end of dose deterioration'.
- Anticholinergic drugs (e.g. benzhexol) may be helpful in controlling tremor and excess salivation that occur in Parkinson's disease.

Lithium

Class: Mood stabilizer

Indications
- Treatment and prophylaxis of mania
- Bipolar affective disorder
- Resistant recurrent depression

Mechanism of action
- Exact mechanism is not fully understood.
- Lithium inhibits secondary messengers in the CNS, possibly through alteration of cyclic AMP and the inositol triphosphate (IP_3) pathway.

Adverse effects
- *Common*: weight gain, nausea, vomiting, diarrhoea, fine tremor
- *Rare*: renal tubular damage, hypothyroidism, muscle weakness, drowsiness, blurred vision, rash, memory impairment (in long term use)

Contraindications
- None
- Caution:
  - Renal impairment (lithium is excreted by the kidneys)
  - Cardiac disease
  - Pregnancy
  - Breast feeding
  - Elderly

Interactions
- *ACE inhibitors*: ACE inhibitors increase the plasma concentration of lithium by reducing its excretion
- *Diuretics*: loop, thiazide and potassium-sparing diuretics increase the plasma concentration of lithium by reducing its excretion
- *NSAIDs*: NSAIDs increase the plasma concentration of lithium by reducing its excretion
- *SSRIs*: SSRIs increase the risk of lithium adverse effects

Route of administration
- Oral

Note
- Thyroid and renal function must be tested prior to and during treatment with lithium because of its nephrotoxic and thyrotoxic effects.
- Lithium has a narrow therapeutic window and so its plasma concentration must be monitored as overdose can be fatal.
- Lithium toxicity manifests as drowsiness, confusion, ataxia, seizures and coma. Management of toxicity includes increasing fluid intake and providing supportive treatment. Haemodialysis should be performed in severe cases.

Phenelzine

Class: Monoamine oxidase inhibitor (MAOI)

Indications
- Depression
- Phobic states

Mechanism of action
- Phenelzine causes non-selective irreversible inhibition of the enzyme monoamine oxidase, which is involved in the metabolism of serotonin, norepinephrine and dopamine. This results in increased concentrations of these neurotransmitters in the brain.
- Monoamine oxidase in the gut wall normally metabolizes tyramine in foodstuffs.

Adverse effects
- *Common*: dizziness, dry mouth, blurred vision, postural hypotension
- *Rare*: hypertensive crisis, jaundice, rash

Contraindications
- Hepatic impairment
- Cerebrovascular disease
- Phaeochromocytoma

Interactions
- ***Carbamazepine***: phenelzine reduces the anticonvulsant effect of carbamazepine
- ***Levodopa and sympathomimetics***: increased risk of a hypertensive crisis (sweating, restlessness, flushing, hyperpyrexia, tremor, convulsions, coma)
- ***Pethidine***: CNS excitation or CNS depression
- ***SSRIs***: increased CNS effects of SSRIs
- ***TCAs***: predisposition to CNS excitation and hypertension
- ***Tyramine-containing foods*** *(e.g. pickled herring, cheese, wine, beer, yeast, chocolate)*: risk of a hypertensive crisis

Route of administration
- Oral

Note
- MAOIs should not be started until at least 2 weeks after a previous MAOI, tricyclic antidepressant or SSRI has been stopped (5 weeks for fluoxetine).
- Other antidepressants should not be started for 2 weeks after treatment with a MAOI has been stopped.
- Patients should carry a warning card, detailing which foods should be avoided.
- Due to its drug and food interactions (especially with tyramine-rich foods) phenelzine is usually a 2nd line drug for the treatment of depression after TCAs and SSRIs.
- Phenelzine is metabolized by acetylation. Slow acetylators (about half the population of Europe and the USA) are more likely to develop adverse effects.

Related drugs
- Isocarboxazid, tranylcypromine

Phenytoin

Class: Anticonvulsant

Indications
- All types of epilepsy except absence seizures
- Trigeminal neuralgia

Mechanism of action
- Phenytoin alters transmembrane movement of Na^+ and K^+ by blocking voltage-gated Na^+ channels.
- It is thought to prevent the spread of epileptic discharges, not the initiation.

Adverse effects
- *Common*: dizziness, headache, confusion, insomnia, nausea, vomiting, coarsening of facial features, hirsutism, acne
- *Rare*: gum hypertrophy, rash, Stevens–Johnson syndrome, blood dyscrasias, drug-induced SLE

Contraindications
- None
- Caution:
  - Hepatic impairment
  - Pregnancy
  - Breast feeding

Interactions
- ***Amiodarone, aspirin, cimetidine, diltiazem and nifedipine***: these drugs increase the plasma concentration of phenytoin
- ***Oral contraceptive pill***: phenytoin decreases the effect of the oral contraceptive pill by increasing its metabolism
- ***Rifampicin***: rifampicin decreases the plasma concentration of phenytoin
- ***Warfarin***: phenytoin increases the metabolism of warfarin
- *Note*: Phenytoin induces hepatic drug-metabolizing enzymes, hence a wide range of further interactions exists

Route of administration
- Oral (epilepsy, trigeminal neuralgia), IV (epilepsy)

Note
- Phenytoin has a narrow therapeutic window and a non-linear relationship between dose and plasma concentration. It therefore requires therapeutic drug monitoring.
- Patients should be advised on how to recognize signs of phenytoin toxicity (mostly CNS effects: tremor, nystagmus, ataxia, dysarthria and convulsions).
- Due to cosmetic adverse effects, phenytoin may be undesirable for use in adolescents.
- Phenytoin is teratogenic and is associated with congenital heart disease and cleft palate/lip.

Related drugs
- Fosphenytoin (a product of phenytoin)

Sodium valproate

Class: Anticonvulsant

Indications
- All types of epilepsy

Mechanism of action
- Sodium valproate increases the GABA content of the brain by inhibiting the enzyme GABA transaminase and preventing GABA re-uptake.
- Sodium valproate also reduces concentrations of aspartate, an excitatory neurotransmitter.
- In addition, it blocks voltage-gated sodium channels.

Adverse effects
- *Common*: nausea, vomiting, weight gain
- *Rare*: hepatic failure, pancreatitis, blood dyscrasias (pancytopenia, thrombocytopenia, leucopenia), sedation, transient hair loss

Contraindications
- Hepatic dysfunction (sodium valproate is metabolized and excreted by the liver)
- Porphyria

Interactions
- *Anticonvulsants*: two or more anticonvulsants given together may lead to enhanced effects, increased sedation or reduced plasma concentrations of either one
- *Neuroleptics*: neuroleptics decrease the anticonvulsant effect of sodium valproate
- *Tricyclic antidepressants*: TCAs decrease the anticonvulsant effect of sodium valproate

Route of administration
- Oral, IV

Note
- Liver function tests should be carried out regularly.
- Sodium valproate is especially useful in children with atonic epilepsy or absence seizures as it has little sedative effect.
- Sodium valproate has fewer adverse effects than most other anticonvulsants.
- Patients should be given an information leaflet describing how to recognize haematological and hepatic adverse effects of sodium valproate.
- Sodium valproate is teratogenic and is associated with congenital abnormalities, including spina bifida.

Sumatriptan

Class: Serotonin (5-HT$_1$) agonist

Indications
- Acute migraine
- Cluster headache (subcutaneous use only)

Mechanism of action
- Sumatriptan selectively stimulates the inhibitory serotonin (5-HT$_1$) receptors in the raphe nucleus of the brain. It thereby maintains vasoconstrictor tone which mainly occurs in the carotid arterial circulation. This is believed to reduce the severity of acute migraine attacks.

Adverse effects
- *Common*: pain at the injection site, flushing, lethargy, tingling
- *Rare*: chest pain, dizziness

Contraindications
- Ischaemic heart disease (sumatriptan produces a small degree of vasoconstriction in coronary vessels)
- Previous myocardial infarction
- Severe hypertension

Interactions
- *Ergotamine*: concomitant use of ergotamine and sumatriptan increases the risk of vasospasm
- *Lithium*: concomitant use of lithium and sumatriptan increases the risk of CNS toxicity
- *MAOIs*: concomitant use of MAOIs and sumatriptan increases the risk of CNS toxicity
- *SSRIs*: concomitant use of SSRIs and sumatriptan increases the risk of CNS toxicity

Route of administration
- Oral, intranasal spray, subcutaneous

Note
- In acute migraine simple analgesics such as paracetamol should be tried first. If these are ineffective, sumatriptan can be used.
- Sumatriptan should be given as soon as possible after the onset of a migraine attack.
- It is more effective if given subcutaneously.
- Sumatriptan is recommended as monotherapy (concomitant use with other antimigraine drugs should be avoided).

Related drugs
- Naratriptan, rizatriptan, zolmitriptan

Temazepam

Class: Benzodiazepine

Indications
- Insomnia
- Premedication before minor surgery

Mechanism of action
- Temazepam binds to GABA receptors in the CNS and thereby facilitates GABA-inhibitory neurotransmission by opening chloride channels. It is thought that this action produces the sedative and anxiolytic effects.

Adverse effects
- *Common*: dependence (with prolonged use)
- *Rare*: seizures, drowsiness, ataxia, anxiety, nightmares, rash, agitation, headache

Contraindications
- Respiratory depression (may be worsened by temazepam)
- Severe hepatic impairment
- Myasthenia gravis
- Sleep apnoea syndrome

Interactions
- *Alcohol*: alcohol enhances the sedative effect of temazepam
- *Cimetidine*: cimetidine inhibits the metabolism of temazepam

Route of administration
- Oral

Note
- Sedative and anxiolytic effects of temazepam last for about 90 min.
- Temazepam should be used short term only to avoid psychological and physical dependence.
- Flumazenil can be used as antidote to temazepam overdose or to reverse its effects.

Related drugs
- Loprazolam, lormetazepam

RHEUMATOLOGY

This chapter provides an account of the management of two important rheumatological conditions followed by a description of relevant individual drugs.

RHEUMATOID ARTHRITIS
- Multidisciplinary team care is important (education, physiotherapy, joint protection, walking aids, orthotics, social services)
- Recommend regular physical exercise

Medical treatment
- First line therapy: paracetamol and NSAIDs for symptom relief (e.g. diclofenac, naproxen)
- Second line therapy: disease-modifying antirheumatic drugs (e.g. sulphasalazine, methotrexate) to slow disease progression
- Third line therapy: alternative DMARDs (e.g. penicillamine, gold, hydroxychloroquine, azathioprine, cyclosporin)
- Corticosteroids can be given for an anti-inflammatory effect:
  - Orally—small doses (e.g. prednisolone) or larger doses in the presence of systemic complications
  - Parenterally—local injection into an inflamed joint, IM long-acting depot injection or large bolus given IV

Surgical treatment
- Surgery may be an option for some patients (e.g. carpal tunnel decompression, synovectomy, tendon repair, arthrodesis, arthroplasty)

GOUT
Acute gout
- In an acute attack give a NSAID (e.g. indomethacin) but *not* aspirin (as it inhibits uric acid excretion)
- If NSAIDs are contraindicated, give colchicine or IM depot injection of corticosteroids

Prevention of gout
- Reduce excessive purine and alcohol intake
- Encourage gradual weight loss, if appropriate
- Consider allopurinol to decrease uric acid synthesis, or a uricosuric drug (e.g. probenecid) to increase urinary uric acid excretion

CORTICOSTEROIDS
Types of corticosteroids
1 Glucocorticoids: beclomethasone, dexamethasone, prednisolone, hydrocortisone
2 Mineralocorticoids: fludrocortisone

Indications
1 Glucocorticoids are mainly used for:
- Suppression of inflammation
- Suppression of the immune system
- Replacement therapy
- Part of chemotherapy (in Hodgkin's lymphoma and acute leukaemia)

2 Mineralocorticoids are mainly used in:
- Replacement therapy

Adverse effects
- Glucocorticoid effects: Cushingoid appearance, osteoporosis, growth suppression, diabetes mellitus, peptic ulcer, cataract, glaucoma, increased risk of infection
- Mineralocorticoid effects: hypokalaemia and hypertension (secondary to sodium and water retention)
- *Note*: Topical use of corticosteroids limits systemic adverse effects

Allopurinol

Class: Anti-gout drug

Indications
- Prophylaxis of gout
- Prophylaxis of uric acid and calcium oxalate renal stones

Mechanism of action
- Allopurinol inhibits the enzyme xanthine oxidase which converts xanthine to uric acid. The excess xanthine is easily excreted as it is more soluble. This decreases uric acid production.

Adverse effects
- *Common*: rash, itching
- *Rare*: hypersensitivity, headache, metallic taste in the mouth, blood disorders, Stevens–Johnson syndrome

Contraindications
- Acute gout attack
- Caution:
  - Renal impairment (allopurinol is renally excreted)

Interactions
- *Ampicillin*: increased risk of skin rash if ampicillin is given with allopurinol
- ***Azathioprine, mercaptopurine***: the effects of these drugs are greatly enhanced by allopurinol, hence they should not be taken together
- *Warfarin*: allopurinol may enhance the effect of warfarin

Route of administration
- Oral

Note
- The risk of a gout attack is increased in the first few weeks of treatment. This can be avoided by taking allopurinol with a NSAID (not aspirin) or colchicine.
- High fluid intake during therapy is recommended (approximately 2 L/day).
- Allopurinol is frequently used to prevent gout in cancer patients receiving chemotherapy.

Azathioprine

Class: Immunosuppressive agent

Indications
- Autoimmune diseases (e.g. rheumatoid arthritis, SLE)
- Prevention of transplant rejection
- Used as a steroid-sparing drug (to allow lower doses of corticosteroids in severe inflammatory conditions)

Mechanism of action
- Azathioprine is metabolized to 6-mercaptopurine in the liver. This metabolite is taken up into cells, where it inhibits DNA synthesis. Azathioprine thus has a cytotoxic effect on dividing cells.

Adverse effects
- *Common*: nausea, vomiting, bone marrow suppression (bleeding, bruising, infections, fatigue)
- *Rare*: alopecia, arthralgia, jaundice

Contraindications
- Pregnancy
- Hypersensitivity

Interactions
- *Allopurinol*: allopurinol inhibits the metabolism of azathioprine, thus increasing the risk of bone marrow suppression

Route of administration
- Oral, IV (very irritant and only rarely used)

Note
- Azathioprine is potentially highly toxic. Close monitoring is required, whereby full blood count is checked weekly for 8 weeks and then every 3 months to exclude bone marrow suppression.
- The standard dose of azathioprine should be reduced in the elderly and in patients with renal or hepatic impairment.

Cyclophosphamide

Class: Alkylating agent (immunosuppressive agent)

Indications
- Malignant tumours (lymphomas, chronic lymphocytic leukaemia, multiple myeloma and solid tumours)
- Vasculitis
- Nephrotic syndrome
- Autoimmune disease (e.g. SLE, rheumatoid arthritis)

Mechanism of action
- Cyclophosphamide is inactive until it undergoes hepatic metabolism.
- It damages the DNA in cells by forming cross-links between strands and by causing base substitution. Consequently, the DNA cannot replicate. This prevents cell division.

Adverse effects
- *Common*: bone marrow suppression, alopecia, and in high dose: nausea, vomiting, anorexia
- *Rare*: haemorrhagic cystitis, infertility in men (with long term use)

Contraindications
- Porphyria

Interactions
- *Suxamethonium*: the effects of suxamethonium are enhanced by cyclophosphamide (alternative muscle relaxants should be used)

Route of administration
- Oral, IV

Note
- To prevent haemorrhagic cystitis, high fluid intake and mesna are recommended. Mesna should be continued for about 24–48 hours after taking cyclophosphamide. It neutralizes acrolein, the toxic metabolite of cyclophosphamide, which damages the bladder.
- As cyclophosphamide acts on the testis, long term treatment may lead to infertility by decreasing the sperm count. This may be irreversible and a discussion regarding sperm storage should therefore be undertaken before therapy.
- Long term use may increase the risk of developing acute myeloid leukaemia.

Cyclosporin

Class: Immunosuppressive agent

Indications
- Autoimmune diseases
- Prevention of transplant rejection
- Prophylaxis and treatment of graft-versus-host disease
- Eczema and psoriasis (when conventional therapy has failed)

Mechanism of action
- Cyclosporin is an immunosuppressive agent directed mainly against T lymphocytes. It prevents their activation and reduces the release of cytokines, especially interleukin-2. This action suppresses cell-mediated immunity and to a lesser extent antibody-mediated immunity.

Adverse effects
- *Common*: nephrotoxicity, hypertension
- *Rare*: hirsutism, gum hypertrophy, convulsions, weakness, hepatic impairment

Contraindications
- Renal disease
- Liver disease

Interactions
- *Note*: Cyclosporin has a wide range of important drug interactions, only some of which are shown below
- *Aminoglycosides, trimethoprim*: these drugs increase plasma cyclosporin levels, thus increasing the risk of nephrotoxicity
- *Carbamazepine, phenytoin, rifampicin*: these drugs reduce the plasma concentration of cyclosporin
- *Diltiazem, nicardipine, verapamil*: these drugs increase the plasma concentration of cyclosporin, thus increasing the risk of nephrotoxicity
- *NSAIDs*: concomitant use of NSAIDs and cyclosporin increases the risk of nephrotoxicity

Route of administration
- Oral, IV

Note
- Unlike other immunosuppresive agents, cyclosporin does not cause bone marrow suppression.
- Therapeutic drug monitoring is required as renal impairment may occur with high doses.
- Some evidence suggests that patients taking cyclosporin are at an increased risk of secondary lymphomas caused by EBV infection. This is believed to be due to impaired immunity.

Methotrexate

Class: Immunosuppressive agent

Indications
- Acute lymphoblastic leukaemia
- Non-Hodgkin's lymphoma
- Choriocarcinoma
- Part of various cancer chemotherapy regimens
- Rheumatoid arthritis
- Psoriasis (when conventional therapy fails)

Mechanism of action
- Methotrexate is a competitive antagonist of the enzyme dihydrofolate reductase, which catalyses the production of tetrahydrofolic acid. This results in decreased production of tetrahydrofolic acid, which is an essential component for synthesis of nucleic material (purines and thymidylic acid). Methotrexate therefore inhibits DNA, RNA and protein synthesis, leading to cell death.

Adverse effects
- *Common*: bone marrow suppression, mucositis (e.g. stomatitis, gingivitis), anorexia, diarrhoea, nausea, vomiting, hepatotoxicity (with prolonged treatment)
- *Rare*: pneumonitis

Contraindications
- Renal impairment (methotrexate is renally excreted)
- Hepatic impairment
- Pregnancy

Interactions
- *Acitretin*: acitretin increases the plasma concentration of methotrexate, thus increasing the risk of hepatotoxicity
- *Cyclosporin*: cyclosporin increases methotrexate toxicity
- *NSAIDs*: NSAIDs increase the risk of methotrexate toxicity by reducing its excretion
- *Probenecid*: probenecid increases the risk of methotrexate toxicity by reducing its excretion

Route of administration
- Oral, IM, IV, intrathecal

Note
- Folinic acid is used to prevent and reverse the toxic effects of methotrexate ('folinic acid rescue').
- Methotrexate has teratogenic effects. Contraceptive precautions are therefore necessary during treatment with methotrexate and 3 months after stopping it.

Penicillamine

Class: Disease-modifying antirheumatic drug (DMARD)

Indications
- Active rheumatoid arthritis (only if disabling or if other drugs have failed)
- Wilson's disease
- Copper poisoning
- Lead poisoning
- Cystinuria

Mechanism of action
- Exact mechanism in rheumatoid arthritis is not fully understood, but penicillamine has immune-modulatory effects by reducing the number of lymphocytes.
- Penicillamine chelates metal ions via its sulphadryl group (hence useful in Wilson's disease and copper/lead poisoning).
- It is thought to form a soluble disulphide complex with cystine (hence useful in cystinuria).

Adverse effects
- *Common*: rash, proteinuria, anorexia, nausea, vomiting
- *Rare*: bone marrow suppression, SLE, pemphigus, fever, mouth ulceration

Contraindications
- Hypersensitivity to penicillin (penicillamine is a degradation product of penicillin)
- SLE

Interactions
- *Iron*: oral iron reduces the absorption of penicillamine

Route of administration
- Oral

Note
- Clinical improvement in rheumatoid arthritis can be expected after 6–12 weeks of treatment and the drug should be stopped if no improvement is evident within 1 year.
- Regular blood and urine tests should be performed to detect any bone marrow suppression or proteinuria.
- Penicillamine should be taken before meals to reduce GI adverse effects.
- Penicillamine should only be prescribed in hospitals by doctors who have experience with this drug.

Prednisolone

Class: Glucocorticoid

Indications
- Anti-inflammatory therapy (e.g. inflammatory bowel disease, asthma, eczema)
- Immunosuppressive therapy (e.g. prevention of transplant rejection, acute leukaemia)
- Glucocorticoid replacement therapy (e.g. congenital adrenal hyperplasia, Addison's disease)

Mechanism of action
- Prednisolone inhibits phospholipase A_2 activity, which is responsible for the production of free arachidonic acid. Arachidonic acid is the precursor for prostaglandin and leukotriene synthesis. Inhibition of this process therefore achieves an anti-inflammatory effect.
- Prednisolone increases gluconeogenesis, redistributes fat to the face, neck and trunk and causes protein breakdown (in tissues such as skin, muscle and bone).
- It decreases B and T lymphocyte response to antigens, thus achieving an immunosuppressive effect.

Adverse effects
- *Common*: bruising, hirsutism, moon-face, hypertension, weight gain/oedema, impaired glucose tolerance, acne, cataract, glaucoma, osteoporosis, peptic ulcer, candida infection (these are subject to dose, route of administration and duration of treatment)
- *Rare*: mood changes (e.g. depression), muscle weakness, reactivation of tuberculosis

Contraindications
- Systemic infection

Interactions
- *Phenytoin*: phenytoin decreases the effect of prednisolone
- *Rifampicin*: rifampicin decreases the effect of prednisolone

Route of administration
- Oral, IM, IV, ear drops, eye drops, rectal

Note
- Patients on prednisolone should be given a steroid card.
- Prednisolone should be withdrawn slowly after long term treatment (> 3 weeks) due to the risk of an acute adrenal crisis (Addisonian crisis).

Related drugs
- Betamethasone, cortisone, dexamethasone, hydrocortisone, prednisone

PAIN MANAGEMENT

GENERAL PRINCIPLES OF PAIN CONTROL
Step 1: non-opioid (e.g. paracetamol, aspirin)
Step 2: weak opioid (e.g. co-proxamol, codeine)
Step 3: strong opioid (e.g. morphine)
• Inadequate analgesia requires a move to the next step
rather than to another drug of similar efficacy

NEURALGIA
• Give a TCA, an anticonvulsant (phenytoin or
carbamazepine) or a membrane-stabilizing drug (e.g.
flecainide)

MUSCLE SPASM PAIN
• Give buscopan (a smooth muscle relaxant) in smooth
muscle spasm (colic)
• Give baclofen (a skeletal muscle relaxant) in muscle spasticity

BONE PAIN
• Give a NSAID (e.g. aspirin)
• Radiotherapy is effective for bone pain caused by
metastases
• Calcitonin or corticosteroids can also be used

RAISED INTRACRANIAL PRESSURE HEADACHE
• Give dexamethasone (a corticosteroid)
• Consider mannitol in severe cases

ALTERNATIVE METHODS OF PAIN CONTROL
• Psychological care (e.g. explanation of pain, reassurance)
• Trans-electrical nervous stimulation (TENS)
• Acupuncture
• Immobilization with collars, splints, corsets, etc. (if
appropriate)
• Nerve block
• Hot or cold applications (e.g. hot water bottle, ice pack)

Drug classes

NON-STEROIDAL ANTI-INFLAMMATORY DRUGS (NSAIDs)
Types of NSAIDs
1 Salicylic acids: aspirin

2 Propionic acids: ibuprofen, naproxen
3 Acetic acids: indomethacin
4 Fenemates: mefenamic acid
5 Pyrazolones: phenylbutazone
6 Phenylacetic acids: diclofenac
7 Oxicams: piroxicam

Indications
- Inflammatory diseases (e.g. rheumatoid arthritis)
- Pain
- Pyrexia

Mechanism of action
- NSAIDs act by reversibly inhibiting COX-1 and COX-2, resulting in decreased prostaglandin production.
- Aspirin acts by irreversibly inhibiting COX-1 and COX-2. It also has an anti-platelet action.
- The desired pharmacological effect of NSAIDs are thought to be due to the inhibition of COX-2.

Adverse effects
- These are mainly related to the inhibition of COX-1 and include:
  - GI disturbances (peptic ulcer, gastritis)
  - Bleeding
  - Bronchoconstriction
  - Renal impairment

OPIATES
Types of opiates
1 Opiate analgesics: morphine, codeine, diamorphine (heroin), dihydrocodeine
2 Non-opiate morphine-like analgesics: pethidine, methadone, dextropropoxyphene, buprenorphine

Indications
- Main indication: pain (morphine or diamorphine are most commonly used in severe pain)
- Other uses:
  - Pulmonary oedema secondary to heart failure (morphine or diamorphine)
  - Diarrhoea (codeine)
  - Cough (codeine or dihydrocodeine)
- Methadone is used to prevent withdrawal symptoms in opiate abusers

Mechanism of action
1 Full agonists: morphine, diamorphine, dihydrocodeine, codeine, pethidine, fentanyl, dextropropoxyphene.
2 Partial agonists: buprenorphine, pentazocine.

Adverse effects
- Respiratory depression (in high doses)
- Constipation
- Nausea and vomiting
- Dependence and tolerance (see Morphine, p. 88)

Opioid antagonists
- These are used to reverse opiate effects (mainly in overdose):
  - Naloxone (rapidly acting)
  - Naltrexone (longer duration of action)

Note
- Codeine is commonly used as a weaker alternative to morphine.
- Opiate antagonists or abrupt withdrawal of an opiate can precipitate a withdrawal syndrome, typically after about 12 hours. It can include symptoms such as yawning, sweating and rhinorrhoea, followed by irritability, insomnia, tremor and gooseflesh ('cold turkey' effect). Symptoms reach a peak 2–3 days after withdrawal and recede after about 1 week. Diarrhoea, vomiting and abdominal cramps can also be present.

Aspirin

Class: NSAID

Indications
- Pain and inflammation
- Prophylaxis of myocardial infarction, ischaemic stroke, transient ischaemic attacks
- Pyrexia

Mechanism of action
- Aspirin irreversibly inhibits the enzymes COX-1 and COX-2. This leads to the inhibition of prostaglandin synthesis and hence to:

    1 a decrease in vascular permeability and vasodilatation (anti-inflammatory effect);

    2 a decrease in sensitization of pain afferents (analgesic effect); and

    3 a decrease in the effect of prostaglandins on the hypothalamus (antipyretic effect).
- Aspirin reduces thromboxane production by platelets, thus inhibiting thrombus formation (anti-platelet effect).

Adverse effects
- *Common*: GI irritation (gastritis, ulcer, bleeding)
- *Rare*: bronchospasm, skin rash, tinnitus, thrombocytopenia, renal impairment

Contraindications
- Children under 12 (aspirin may cause Reye's syndrome) except in juvenile arthritis
- Active peptic ulcer
- Gout
- Bleeding disorders (e.g. haemophilia)
- Breast feeding
- Pregnancy at term

Interactions
- *Methotrexate*: aspirin increases the risk of toxic effects of methotrexate
- **Warfarin**: concomitant use of aspirin and warfarin increases the risk of bleeding

Route of administration
- Oral, rectal

Note
- The risk of gastric irritation can be slightly reduced by taking aspirin with food or by using the enteric-coated form.
- In high doses aspirin can lead to salicylate intoxication (dizziness, tinnitus, deafness).
- Aspirin is associated with Reye's syndrome in children under 12 years of age (a childhood condition characterized by encephalitis and liver failure). Paracetamol is thus the preferred option in this age group.

Related drugs
- NSAIDs: diclofenac, ibuprofen
- Antiplatelet drugs: clopidogrel, dipyridamole

Co-proxamol

Class: Compound analgesic (paracetamol + dextropropoxyphene)

Indications
- Moderate pain

Mechanism of action
- The paracetamol component inhibits production of chemical mediators that cause pain (see Paracetamol, p. 89).
- The dextropropoxyphene component acts by binding to opiate receptors in the CNS to decrease pain (see Morphine, p. 88).

Adverse effects
- *Common*: nausea, vomiting, constipation, drowsiness
- *Rare*: rash, euphoria

Contraindications
- None
- Caution:
  - Asthma
  - Chronic respiratory disease
  - Elderly (reduce the dose)
  - Therapy with hepatic enzyme-inducing drugs (e.g. anticonvulsants, alcohol) as the risk of hepatotoxicity is increased

Interactions
- See Paracetamol, Morphine (pp. 88 and 89)

Route of administration
- Oral

Note
- If co-proxamol is prescribed long term, tolerance and dependence may develop due to dextropropoxyphene (the opiate component).
- Co-proxamol overdose can be hazardous as dextropropoxyphene may cause respiratory depression and paracetamol may lead to liver damage.
- There is no evidence that co-proxamol is superior to paracetamol in short term use.

Related drugs
- Co-codamol (paracetamol + codeine phosphate), co-dydramol (paracetamol + dihydrocodeine)

Morphine

Class: Opioid analgesic

Indications
- Severe pain (e.g. myocardial infarction, perioperative analgesia, pain in terminal care)
- Acute pulmonary oedema due to heart failure
- Intractable cough in terminal care

Mechanism of action
- Morphine mimics endogenous opioids by acting on μ, δ and κ opioid receptors in the dorsal horn, periaqueductal grey matter and midline raphe nuclei.

Adverse effects
- *Common*: nausea, vomiting, drowsiness, constipation, dry mouth, dizziness, respiratory depression in overdose
- *Rare*: dependence, hallucinations, difficulty with micturition, urticaria, headache, palpitations, mood changes

Contraindications
- Severe respiratory disease (e.g. COPD)
- Raised intracranial pressure (morphine interferes with neurological assessment)
- Head injury (morphine interferes with neurological assessment)
- Undiagnosed acute abdomen
- Acute alcohol intoxication
- Hepatic failure

Interactions
- *Hypnotics*: morphine enhances the sedative effect of hypnotics

Route of administration
- IM, IV, oral, sublingual, rectal, subcutaneous

Note
- The effects of morphine can be reversed with naloxone, a rapidly acting opioid antagonist.
- Tolerance to morphine begins to emerge after about 2 weeks of continuous treatment. Subsequently, the dose should be increased.
- Dependence on morphine develops gradually. It is very uncommon when used to treat pain.
- Abrupt withdrawal of morphine results in a withdrawal syndrome (myalgia, sweating, yawning).

Related drugs
- Codeine, diamorphine, dihydrocodeine

Paracetamol

Class: Non-opiate analgesic and antipyretic

Indications
- Mild to moderate pain
- Pyrexia (especially in children)

Mechanism of action
- Paracetamol is a weak inhibitor of the enzyme cyclo-oxygenase which is responsible for the production of prostaglandins and thromboxane. This may contribute to the mechanism of action but it is not clearly understood.
- Paracetamol does not exert any anti-platelet action (unlike aspirin). It has tissue specificity for the CNS, resulting in its antipyretic and analgesic effects with little anti-inflammatory action.

Adverse effects
- *Rare*: rash, blood dyscrasias; hepatic necrosis and renal failure in overdose

Contraindications
- None
- Caution:
  - Hepatic impairment
  - Renal impairment
  - Chronic alcohol abuse

Interactions
- No serious interactions

Route of administration
- Oral, rectal

Note
- Paracetamol is used in patients who are intolerant of aspirin.
- Paracetamol is commonly used in children as it is not associated with Reye's syndrome (unlike aspirin).
- It does not cause gastric irritation and is therefore preferred to aspirin for pain relief, especially in the elderly.
- Paracetamol is effective in the relief of musculoskeletal pain. In visceral pain opiates are the preferred treatment.
- Toxic metabolites of paracetamol are generated more rapidly when administered with drugs which induce hepatic enzymes (e.g. rifampicin).
- *N*-acetylcysteine is an effective antidote in paracetamol overdose.

Pethidine

Class: Opioid analgesic

Indications
- Analgesia in labour
- Moderate to severe pain

Mechanism of action
- Pethidine acts by stimulating opioid μ, δ and κ receptors in the dorsal horn of the spinal cord, the peri-aqueductal grey matter and in the midline raphe nuclei.
- It creates a sense of euphoria, which contributes to the analgesic effect by reducing anxiety and stress.
- Owing to its lipid-solubility, pethidine has a rapid onset of action.

Adverse effects
- *Common*: dizziness, nausea, vomiting, drowsiness, confusion, constipation
- *Rare*: shortness of breath, convulsions in overdose

Contraindications
- Severe renal impairment
- Respiratory failure
- Alcoholism

Interactions
- *MAOIs*: MAOIs given with pethidine can cause CNS excitation or CNS depression

Route of administration
- Oral, IM, IV, subcutaneous

Note
- Pethidine is used in labour as adverse effects on the baby are less pronounced than with other opiates (due to its short half-life of 2–4 hours) and because it does not inhibit uterine contractions. Pethidine may, however, cause respiratory depression in the neonate.
- Larger doses of pethidine are required if given orally due to extensive first pass metabolism.
- Pethidine does not cause pupillary constriction in overdose.
- Naloxone is an effective antidote in pethidine overdose.
- Norpethidine, a metabolite of pethidine, may accumulate and cause convulsions by stimulating the CNS. This is more likely in renal impairment.

Related drugs
- Buprenorphine, dextropropoxyphene, methadone

INFECTION

This chapter provides an overview of antimicrobial treatments (antibiotics, antifungal and antiviral agents). We have included an outline of the treatment of some specific infections and common skin conditions. This is followed by a detailed account of commonly used antimicrobial agents.

ANTIBIOTICS

Antibiotics work by acting on microbial components which are either absent or radically different in human cells (i.e. selective toxicity). There are three main mechanisms by which they arrest microbial growth, as detailed below.

1 Inhibition of cell wall synthesis:
   - Penicillins
     - Benzylpenicillin
     - Broad-spectrum penicillins: amoxycillin, ampicillin
     - Antipseudomonal penicillins: azlocillin, piperacillin, ticarcillin
     - β-lactamase-resistant penicillins: cloxacillin, flucloxacillin
   - Cephalosporins
     - First generation: cephalexin, cephradine
     - Second generation: cefuroxime
     - Third generation: cefotaxime, ceftriaxone
   - Glycopeptides
     - Teicoplanin, vancomycin
   - Carbapenems
     - Imipenem
   - Monobactams
     - Aztreonam

2 Inhibition of nucleic acid synthesis
   - Quinolones: cinoxacin, ciprofloxacin, nalidixic acid, norfloxacin
   - Trimethoprim
   - Sulphonamides: sulphamethoxazole
   - Metronidazole
   - Nitrofurantoin
   - Rifampicin

3 Inhibition of protein synthesis
   (a) By acting on the bacterial 30S ribosomal subunit:
      - Aminoglycosides: amikacin, gentamicin, kanamycin, neomycin, tobramycin
      - Tetracyclines: doxycycline, minocycline, oxytetracycline, tetracycline
   (b) By acting on the bacterial 50S ribosomal subunit:
      - Macrolides: azithromycin, clarithromycin, erythromycin
      - Clindamycin
      - Chloramphenicol
      - Fusidic acid

The following table shows some common pathogens and antibiotics that can be used to treat them. It should be noted that resistance to many antibiotics is emerging and the regimens shown here are subject to change.

Pathogen	Treatment of choice
Anaerobes	Metronidazole
Bordetella pertussis	Erythromycin
Chlamydia trachomatis	Doxycycline
Clostridium difficile	Stop any antibiotics and give oral metronidazole or vancomycin
Enterococcus spp.	Amoxycillin/ampicillin + gentamicin
Escherichia coli	Ceftriaxone
Haemophilus influenzae	Amoxycillin (only if β-lactamase negative)
Legionella	Erythromycin
Listeria monocytogenes	Ampicillin (+ gentamicin)
Mycobacterium tuberculosis	Rifampicin + isoniazid + pyrazinamide (+ ethambutol)
Mycoplasma pneumoniae	Erythromycin or tetracycline
Neisseria gonorrhoeae	Penicillin
Neisseria meningitidis	Penicillin
Pseudomonas aeruginosa	Antipseudomonal penicillin + aminoglycoside
Staphylococcus spp.	Flucloxacillin *or* vancomycin + gentamicin *or* fusidic acid
Streptococcus spp.	Penicillins or cephalosporins (erythromycin in penicillin allergy)

ANTIFUNGALS
Fungal infections (termed mycoses) are difficult to treat. They usually involve the skin, nails or mucous membranes. Systemic fungal infections usually occur in immuno-compromised individuals. There are four main classes of antifungal drugs:
1 Polyenes
  • These act by forming pores in the fungal membrane, leading to cell death (e.g. amphotericin, nystatin)
2 Imidazoles
  • These act by inhibiting synthesis of lipids in the fungal cell membrane (e.g. clotrimazole, ketoconazole)
3 Triazoles
  • These act by a mechanism similar to the imidazoles (e.g. fluconazole, itraconazole)
4 Others
  • These include flucytosine, griseofulvin and terbinafine

ANTIVIRALS

Viruses, which live and replicate inside human cells, make use of the metabolic pathways of the host cell. It is thus very difficult to direct treatment selectively against the virus without in some way adversely affecting the patient.

- There are three main mechanisms by which antiviral agents work:
    1 Inhibition of viral nucleic acid synthesis (e.g. aciclovir, ganciclovir, ribavirin, zidovudine)
    2 Inhibition of penetration into host cell (e.g. amantadine)
    3 Antiviral activity (e.g. interferons)

BACTERIAL MENINGITIS

Neonates
- Most likely organisms are:
    - Group B streptococci—treat with IV benzylpenicillin + IV gentamicin
    - *Escherichia coli*—treat with IV cefotaxime
    - *Listeria monocytogenes*—treat with IV ampicillin
- Blind therapy—IV penicillin + IV gentamicin

Infant/toddler
- Most likely organisms are:
    - *Haemophilus influenzae*—treat with IV cefotaxime (incidence decreasing due to Hib vaccine)
    - *Neisseria meningitidis*—treat with IV benzylpenicillin or IV cefotaxime
    - *Streptococcus pneumoniae*—treat with IV cefotaxime or IV benzylpenicillin
- Blind therapy—IV cefotaxime *or* IV chloramphenicol + IV benzylpenicillin

From age 4 onwards
- Most likely organisms are:
    - *Neisseria meningitidis*—treat with IV benzylpenicillin or IV cefotaxime
    - *Streptococcus pneumoniae*—treat with IV cefotaxime or IV benzylpenicillin
- Blind therapy—IV chloramphenicol + IV benzylpenicillin *or* IV cefotaxime

Note
- Corticosteroids may be given to decrease the risk of complications of meningitis (e.g. deafness, cerebral oedema).
- Rifampicin is given to contacts such as family members for a period of 48 hours to prevent spread of meningitis caused by *Neisseria meningitidis* or *Haemophilus influenzae*.
- Fluids may be given if required.

TUBERCULOUS MENINGITIS
• Anti-tuberculous therapy (rifampicin, pyrazinamide, isoniazid) for 9 months

VIRAL MENINGITIS
• Many viruses may cause meningitis (e.g. enteroviruses, mumps)
• Treatment is supportive (e.g. bed rest, pain relief) as viral meningitis is a self-limiting condition

OTITIS MEDIA
• Common causative organisms are *Streptococcus pneumoniae* and *Haemophilus influenzae*
• In acute otitis media, give IV amoxycillin (in severe cases give IV benzylpenicillin followed by oral penicillin)
• In chronic otitis media consider myringotomy and grommet insertion

THROAT INFECTIONS
• Viral infections are the commonest cause of sore throat and should not be treated with antibiotics
• Most common bacterial cause is *Streptococcus pyogenes*, for which oral penicillin or a cephalosporin can be given for 10 days to prevent complications such as rheumatic fever or glomerulonephritis (give erythromycin in penicillin allergy)

CONJUNCTIVITIS
• In allergic conjunctivitis give sodium cromoglycate or antihistamine eye drops
• In bacterial conjunctivitis (mostly caused by staphylococci) give chloramphenicol or gentamicin eye drops
• In viral conjunctivitis caused by herpes simplex give aciclovir eye drops

INFECTIVE ENDOCARDITIS
Prophylaxis of endocarditis
• This is necessary in patients with cardiac abnormalities (e.g. congenital defects, artificial heart valves) and other high-risk groups undergoing the following:
  1 Dental procedures under local or no anaesthetic:
    • Give oral amoxycillin 1 hour before the dental procedure (oral clindamycin if allergic to penicillin or if penicillin was given in the past month)
    • Add gentamicin if the patient has had previous endocarditis
  2 Surgery or GI/urinary tract instrumentation:
    • Give IV amoxycillin + IV gentamicin

Treatment of endocarditis
- Treatment depends on organism susceptibility and usually lasts for about 2–4 weeks
- Streptococcal endocarditis: give IV benzylpenicillin + IV gentamicin
- Staphylococcal endocarditis: give IV flucloxacillin + IV gentamicin
- Enterococcal endocarditis: give IV amoxycillin + IV gentamicin

PNEUMONIA
General management
- Bed rest
- Pain relief
- Oral/IV fluids
- 60% oxygen (24% in COPD)
- IV antibiotics (see below)

Community-acquired pneumonia
- Mostly caused by *Streptococcus pneumoniae*, followed by *Mycoplasma pneumoniae*
- Treat with amoxycillin or benzylpenicillin (erythromycin in penicillin allergy)
- Add flucloxacillin if staphylococcal infection is suspected

Hospital-acquired pneumonia
- Mostly caused by *Pseudomonas aeruginosa*, *Klebsiella*, *Staphylococcus aureus*, *Escherichia coli*
- Treat with a cephalosporin (e.g. cefotaxime) + aminoglycoside (e.g. gentamicin)
- Add metronidazole if anaerobic infection is suspected (e.g. aspiration pneumonia)

Atypical pneumonia
- Mostly caused by *Mycoplasma pneumoniae*, *Chlamydia pneumoniae*, *Chlamydia psittaci*, *Coxiella burnetii* and *Legionella* infections
- Treat with erythromycin or tetracycline

Blind therapy
- Treat with erythromycin + *either* cefuroxime *or* cefotaxime
- Add flucloxacillin if staphylococcal infection is suspected

URINARY TRACT INFECTIONS
- UTIs can be classified into infection of the kidney (pyelonephritis), bladder (cystitis) and urethra (urethritis)
- The commonest cause is *Escherichia coli*

Principles of management
- Increase fluid intake

- Analgesia
- Antibiotics (see below)

Children
- Give oral trimethoprim for 7 days and then as prophylaxis until the cause has been investigated
- Investigate for any underlying structural abnormalities (e.g. ureteric obstruction) and vesicoureteric reflux whilst maintaining therapy with trimethoprim
- In cases of vesicoureteric reflux, consider long term prophylactic antibiotics (e.g. trimethoprim, nitrofurantoin) to prevent renal scarring

Adults
- Give trimethoprim or amoxycillin or a cephalosporin (e.g. cefuroxime) or nitrofurantoin (do not give trimethoprim in pregnancy)
- Usually a single dose or a short course of antibiotic is sufficient
- Males should always be investigated for underlying pathology (e.g. obstruction due to prostate enlargement or calculi)

PELVIC INFLAMMATORY DISEASE
- Commonest cause is *Chlamydia trachomatis* followed by *Neisseria gonorrhoeae*
- Treat promptly to prevent complications (e.g. infertility, ectopic pregnancy): give doxycycline and metronidazole for 7–14 days (remove IUCD if present)
- Give analgesia if required (many patients are asymptomatic)
- Consider laparoscopy if antibiotics are ineffective (diagnosis of PID may be incorrect)
- Recommend barrier contraception or abstinence until recovery is made to prevent spread of the infection
- Contact screening is recommended

SEPTICAEMIA
- Take blood cultures before starting antibiotic therapy
- Give blind therapy until blood culture results are available: IV gentamicin + *either* IV amoxycillin *or* an IV cephalosporin (e.g. cefotaxime)
- When results are available, adapt antibiotic therapy if necessary
- Investigate the source in the body and treat accordingly

TUBERCULOSIS
Phase 1: rifampicin + isoniazid + pyrazinamide for 2 months
Phase 2: rifampicin + isoniazid for 4 months

- In cases of suspected isoniazid resistance, ethambutol may be given
- Give pyridoxine (vitamin B$_6$) throughout treatment as isoniazid can cause vitamin B$_6$ deficiency

SKIN CONDITIONS

Impetigo
- Usually caused by staphylococci and Group A streptococci
- Treat topically with fusidic acid or mupirocin
- Widespread infection should be treated with oral flucloxacillin or erythromycin

Erysipelas
- Usually caused by group A streptococci
- Treat systemically with penicillin

Cellulitis
- Usually caused by a combination of staphylococci and group A streptococci
- Treat systemically with penicillin and flucloxacillin

Acne
1 Topical treatment (for mild or moderate acne and as an adjunct to severe acne):
   - Keratolytic agents—benzoyl peroxide, salicylic acid
   - Antibiotics—erythromycin, clindamycin
   - Retinoids—isotretinoin
2 Systemic treatment (for moderate to severe acne):
   - Antibiotics (e.g. tetracycline, doxycycline) for a minimum of 6 months
   - Hormonal tretment (cyproterone acetate + ethinyloestradiol)—only in females
   - Retinoids—isotretinoin

Rosacea
- Avoid precipitants (e.g. coffee, alcohol, spicy foods)
- Give long term oral tetracycline or topical metronidazole
- Treat any complications (e.g. rhinophyma, blepharitis, conjunctivitis)

Psoriasis
- Topical and systemic agents (as shown below) can be used in various combinations and should be tailored to the individual:
   1 Topical treatment (for mild to moderate psoriasis):
      - Emollients
      - Coal tar
      - Corticosteroids (e.g. beclomethasone)
      - Dithranol
      - Vitamin D analogues (e.g. calcipotriol)
      - UVB radiation

2 Systemic treatment (for moderate to severe psoriasis):
  - Psoralen with ultraviolet A radiation (PUVA)
  - Acitretin
  - Methotrexate
  - Cyclosporin
  - Hydroxyurea

Eczema
- Avoid irritants if possible (e.g. bleaches, soaps, detergents)
- Topical and systemic agents (as shown below) can be used in various combinations and should be tailored to the individual:
  1 Topical treatment (for mild to moderate eczema):
    - Emollients—used on skin and in bath water
    - Coal tar
    - Corticosteroids
    - Antibiotics for superimposed infections
  2 Systemic treatment (for moderate to severe eczema):
    - Corticosteroids or other immunosuppressive agents (e.g. cyclosporin)
    - Antihistamines (to reduce itching)
    - Antibiotics for superimposed infections

Aciclovir

Class: Antiviral drug

Indications
- Infections caused by α herpes viruses (herpes simplex types 1 and 2, varicella-zoster virus)

Mechanism of action
- Aciclovir is selectively taken up by virus-infected cells. It is preferentially phosphorylated by herpes virus-encoded thymidine kinase to aciclovir monophosphate. This is then converted to aciclovir triphosphate by cellular phosphokinases. Aciclovir triphosphate is incorporated into herpes DNA and acts as a chain terminator.

Adverse effects
- *Rare*: rash (topical lotion); nausea, vomiting, headache (oral route); renal impairment (if given too quickly IV); confusion, hallucinations (IV route); inflammation at the drip site (if there is leakage into tissues)

Contraindications
- None
- Not licensed in pregnancy and breast feeding, but commonly used

Interactions
- *Probenecid*: probenecid increases the plasma concentration of aciclovir by decreasing its excretion (this does not apply to topical preparations)

Route of administration
- Oral, topical, IV

Note
- Aciclovir is prescribed for herpes simplex types 1 and 2 infections (genital herpes, cold sores, encephalitis, eye infections). It is also used to treat shingles (caused by varicella-zoster virus).
- If encephalitis is suspected IV aciclovir should be given immediately.
- Ganciclovir is more effective than aciclovir in the treatment of CMV and EBV infections (but is more toxic).
- In aciclovir resistance foscarnet or cidofovir should be used.

Related drugs
- Famciclovir, valaciclovir

Amoxycillin

Class: β-lactam antibiotic

Indications
- Wide range of infections caused by Gram positive (e.g. *Streptococcus* spp., *Staphylococcus* spp.) and Gram negative (e.g. *Haemophilus influenzae*) bacteria
- Part of *Helicobacter pylori* eradication therapy
- Prophylaxis of infectious endocarditis prior to dental/surgical procedures

Mechanism of action
- Amoxycillin is a broad-spectrum bactericidal antibiotic.
- It inhibits bacterial cell wall synthesis by preventing formation of cross-links between peptidoglycan chains which constitute the cell wall.

Adverse effects
- *Common*: skin rash, diarrhoea, nausea, vomiting, candida vaginitis
- *Rare*: anaphylactic shock

Contraindications
- Penicillin hypersensitivity

Interactions
- ***Oral contraceptive pill***: amoxycillin reduces the effectiveness of the pill, hence other contraceptive precautions must be taken during treatment
- *Probenecid*: probenecid decreases the excretion of amoxycillin

Route of administration
- Oral, IM, IV

Note
- Certain strains of bacteria produce the enzyme β-lactamase which inactivates amoxycillin. To prevent this amoxycillin can be usefully combined with clavulanic acid (known as co-amoxiclav).
- Amoxycillin characteristically causes a rash in patients who have infectious mononucleosis.

Related drugs
- Ampicillin

Benzylpenicillin

Class: β-lactam antibiotic

Indications
- Infections caused by *Streptococcus* spp., *Neisseria meningitidis* and *Neisseria gonorrhoeae*
- Also used in infections caused by *Treponema pallidum*, *Corynebacterium diphtheriae*, *Clostridium tetani* and other susceptible organisms

Mechanism of action
- Benzylpenicillin is a bactericidal antibiotic.
- It inhibits bacterial cell wall synthesis by preventing formation of cross-links between peptidoglycan chains which constitute the cell wall.

Adverse effects
- *Common*: rash, diarrhoea
- *Rare*: anaphylactic shock; bone marrow suppression and convulsions in high doses

Contraindications
- Penicillin hypersensitivity

Interactions
- *Indomethacin*: indomethacin decreases the excretion of benzylpenicillin
- *Probenecid*: probenecid decreases the excretion of benzylpenicillin (a useful interaction which allows dose reduction of penicillin)

Route of administration
- IV, IM

Note
- Benzylpenicillin is inactivated by the enzyme β-lactamase, which is produced by many organisms (e.g. *Staphylococcus* spp., some strains of *Escherichia coli* and *Pseudomonas*). β-lactamase-resistant penicillins (e.g. flucloxacillin) or antipseudomonal penicillins (e.g. ticarcillin) can be used against these organisms.
- Phenoxymethylpenicillin (penicillin V) is the oral equivalent of benzylpenicillin. It has poor bioavailability.
- Benzylpenicillin IM or IV should be given immediately if meningococcal meningitis is suspected.
- In cases of penicillin allergy erythromycin can be given.

Cefuroxime

Class: 2nd generation cephalosporin (β-lactam antibiotic)

Indications
- Infections caused by Gram positive and Gram negative organisms (e.g. *Streptococcus* spp., *Staphylococcus* spp., *Escherichia coli*, *Haemophilus influenzae*)

Mechanism of action
- Cefuroxime inhibits bacterial cell wall synthesis by preventing formation of cross-links between peptidoglycan chains, which constitute the bacterial cell wall.

Adverse effects
- *Common*: diarrhoea
- *Rare*: thrombophlebitis (at the site of IV injection), haemorrhage (cefuroxime interferes with clotting factors), hypersensitivity, nausea, vomiting, antibiotic-associated colitis

Contraindications
- Hypersensitivity
- Porphyria
- Caution:
  - Penicillin allergy (about 10% of patients who are allergic to penicillin will have an allergic reaction to cephalosporins)

Interactions
- *Probenecid*: probenecid increases the plasma concentration of cefuroxime by decreasing its excretion
- *Warfarin*: cefuroxime possibly enhances the anticoagulant effect of warfarin

Route of administration
- Oral, IM, IV, eye drops

Note
- Currently there are three generations of cephalosporins available:
  - First generation (cephradine),
  - Second generation (cefuroxime, cephamandole) and
  - Third generation (cefotaxime, ceftriaxone, ceftazidime).
- First and second generation cephalosporins are used against both Gram negative and Gram positive organisms.
- Third generation cephalosporins are less toxic, more efficacious and more specific towards Gram negative organisms.

Ciprofloxacin

Class: Quinolone antibiotic

Indications
- Mainly Gram negative infections (e.g. *Salmonella* spp., *Pseudomonas* spp., *Campylobacter* spp., *Neisseria* spp., *Escherichia coli*, *Haemophilus influenzae*)
- Some Gram positive infections

Mechanism of action
- Ciprofloxacin is a broad-spectrum bactericidal antibiotic.
- It inhibits the activity of the bacterial enzyme DNA gyrase, which is necessary for coiling and replication of bacterial DNA. Human cells do not contain DNA gyrase.

Adverse effects
- *Common*: nausea, vomiting, abdominal pain, diarrhoea
- *Rare*: insomnia, confusion, convulsions

Contraindications
- Pregnancy
- Children (animal studies have shown damage to cartilage)
- Caution:
  - Epilepsy (ciprofloxacin lowers the seizure threshold)

Interactions
- ***Cyclosporin***: concomitant use of ciprofloxacin and cyclosporin increases the risk of nephrotoxicity
- ***Theophylline***: the risk of convulsions is increased if ciprofloxacin is combined with theophylline
- ***Warfarin***: ciprofloxacin enhances the anticoagulant effect of warfarin

Route of administration
- Oral, IV, eye drops

Note
- Ciprofloxacin is clinically used in respiratory tract, urinary tract and GI tract infections. It is also used in gonorrhoea and septicaemia.
- Ciprofloxacin is mainly used to treat bacterial infections that are resistant to other commonly used antibiotics. Bacteria may become resistant to quinolones due to a mutation in their DNA gyrase.

Related drugs
- Grepafloxacin, levofloxacin, nalidixic acid, norfloxacin, ofloxacin

Erythromycin

Class: Macrolide antibiotic

Indications
- Alternative to penicillin in penicillin allergy
- Infections caused by Gram positive and some Gram negative bacteria
- *Mycoplasma pneumoniae*, *Legionella pneumophila* and *Chlamydia* infections
- Acne
- Rosacea

Mechanism of action
- Erythromycin is a broad-spectrum bacteriostatic antibiotic.
- It inhibits bacterial protein synthesis by reversibly binding to the 50S subunit of the bacterial ribosome.

Adverse effects
- *Common*: nausea, vomiting, diarrhoea, rash, phlebitis (when injected into a peripheral vein)
- *Rare*: reversible hearing loss (with high doses), cholestatic jaundice

Contraindications
- Liver disease

Interactions
- *Antihistamines*: erythromycin inhibits the metabolism of astemizole and terfenadine, thus increasing the risk of cardiac dysrhythmias
- *Cyclosporin*: erythromycin increases the plasma concentration of cyclosporin
- *Digoxin*: the effects of digoxin are enhanced by erythromycin
- *Theophylline*: erythromycin increases the plasma concentration of theophylline
- *Warfarin*: erythromycin enhances the anticoagulant effect of warfarin
- *Note*: Erythromycin inhibits hepatic drug-metabolizing enzymes, hence a wide range of further interactions exists

Route of administration
- Oral, IV infusion

Note
- A course of erythromycin for longer than 14 days increases the risk of hepatic damage.

Related drugs
- Azithromycin, clarithromycin (both have fewer GI adverse effects)

Flucloxacillin

Class: β-lactam antibiotic

Indications
- *Staphylococcus aureus* infections (e.g. impetigo, cellulitis)

Mechanism of action
- Flucloxacillin is a narrow-spectrum bactericidal antibiotic.
- It inhibits bacterial cell wall synthesis by preventing cross-linking between peptidoglycan chains which constitute the bacterial cell wall.

Adverse effects
- *Common*: hypersensitivity (rash, urticaria, fever)
- *Rare*: anaphylaxis

Contraindications
- Penicillin allergy

Interactions
- *COC pill*: flucloxacillin can reduce the contraceptive effect

Route of administration
- Oral, IM, IV

Note
- Unlike other penicillins, flucloxacillin is resistant to staphylococcal β-lactamase. This enzyme cleaves the β-lactam ring rendering non-resistant penicillins inactive.
- Flucloxacillin-resistant strains of *Staphylococcus aureus* (i.e. MRSA) have emerged in many hospitals. Therapy with vancomycin or teicoplanin is usually indicated for these organisms.
- Patients taking both the COC pill and flucloxacillin must be informed of the reduced contraceptive effect.

Related drugs
- Cloxacillin

Gentamicin

Class: Aminoglycoside antibiotic

Indications
- Serious infections caused by aerobic Gram negative bacteria
- Staphylococcal infections

Mechanism of action
- Gentamicin is bactericidal.
- Gentamicin inhibits bacterial protein synthesis by binding irreversibly to the 30S subunit of the bacterial ribosome.

Adverse effects
- *Common*: hypersensitivity reaction
- *Rare*: nephrotoxicity, ototoxicity (causes 8th cranial nerve damage)

Contraindications
- Myasthenia gravis
- Pregnancy (gentamicin crosses the placenta and can damage the fetal 8th cranial nerve)

Interactions
- *Cyclosporin*: cyclosporin potentiates nephrotoxic effects of gentamicin
- *Cytotoxics*: cytotoxics potentiate nephrotoxic and ototoxic effects of gentamicin
- *Loop diuretics*: loop diuretics potentiate ototoxic and nephrotoxic effects of gentamicin
- *Neostigmine, pyridostigmine*: gentamicin antagonizes the effects of these drugs

Route of administration
- IV, IM, topical, intrathecal

Note
- Gentamicin is not usually given over periods longer than 10 days because of potential ototoxicity and nephrotoxicity.
- Gentamicin has a narrow therapeutic window, so therapeutic drug monitoring is essential.
- Gentamicin is usually combined with penicillin and/or metronidazole in blind therapy for serious infections.
- Amikacin can be used to treat serious infections caused by Gram negative bacilli that are resistant to gentamicin.
- Gentamicin can cause grey baby syndrome in neonates. The grey skin discoloration is a consequence of tissue hypoperfusion and shock.

Related drugs
- Amikacin, kanamycin, neomycin, netilmicin, tobramycin

Metronidazole

Class: Antibiotic

Indications
- Anaerobic and protozoal infections
- Part of *Helicobacter pylori* eradication therapy
- Rosacea
- Pseudomembranous colitis

Mechanism of action
- Metronidazole is a bactericidal antibiotic.
- It is broken down into toxic compounds within microbes that possess anaerobic or microaerophilic metabolism. These toxic compounds kill the microbes by interfering with their nucleic acid function and synthesis.

Adverse effects
- *Common*: nausea, vomiting, anorexia, diarrhoea
- *Rare*: anaphylaxis, drowsiness, headache, dizziness, metallic taste in the mouth

Contraindications
- None
- Caution:
  - Pregnancy
  - Breast feeding
  - Hepatic impairment

Interactions
- *Alcohol*: alcohol causes disulfiram-like reaction with metronidazole (flushing, abdominal pain, hypotension)
- *Phenytoin*: metronidazole increases the plasma concentration of phenytoin by inhibiting its metabolism
- *Warfarin*: metronidazole enhances the anticoagulant effect of warfarin by inhibiting its metabolism

Route of administration
- Oral, IV, rectal

Note
- Therapeutic drug monitoring is advised for treatment exceeding 10 days.
- Metronidazole is commonly used to treat dental infections as these are mostly caused by anaerobes.

Related drugs
- Tinidazole (longer duration of action)

Rifampicin

Class: Antituberculous agent

Indications
- Tuberculosis
- Leprosy
- Prophylaxis against meningococcal meningitis and *Haemophilus influenzae* type b infection in contacts of cases

Mechanism of action
- Rifampicin inhibits the DNA-dependant RNA polymerase isoenzyme in bacteria (but not in human cells) and is thus bactericidal.

Adverse effects
- *Common*: disturbance of LFTs, pink-coloured tears and urine
- *Rare*: hepatitis, rash, thrombocytopenia, nausea, vomiting, anorexia, flu-like illness

Contraindications
- Jaundice
- Porphyria

Interactions
- *Calcium channel blockers, carbamazepine, corticosteroids and phenytoin*: rifampicin accelerates the metabolism of these drugs, thus reducing their effects
- ***Oestrogens and progestogens***: rifampicin accelerates the metabolism of the COC pill, thus reducing the contraceptive effect
- *Warfarin*: rifampicin increases the metabolism of warfarin, thus decreasing its effect
- *Note*: Rifampicin induces hepatic drug-metabolizing enzymes, hence a wide range of further interactions exists

Route of administration
- Oral, IV

Note
- Resistance to rifampicin can develop rapidly if it is used alone. Therefore it is usually given in combination with ethambutol, pyrazinamide and isoniazid in patients with tuberculosis.
- Liver function tests should be carried out before treatment. The patient should be told how to recognize signs of liver dysfunction. If these occur, LFTs should be repeated.
- Compliance may be difficult, as treatment for tuberculosis lasts for 6 months.

Tetracycline

Class: Tetracycline antibiotic

Indications
- Infections caused by *Coxiella burnetii*, *Mycoplasma* spp., *Leptospira ictohaemorrhagiae*, *Chlamydia* spp., *Rickettsia* spp., *Borrellia burgdorferi* and other susceptible organisms
- Acne

Mechanism of action
- Tetracycline is bacteriostatic.
- It undergoes selective uptake into bacterial cells and binds reversibly to the 30S subunit of the ribosome. This disrupts protein synthesis by interfering with translation.

Adverse effects
- *Common*: nausea, vomiting, diarrhoea
- *Rare*: acute renal failure

Contraindications
- Children
- Pregnancy
- Breast feeding
- Renal impairment
- SLE

Interactions
- *Antacids*: antacids decrease the absorption of tetracycline
- *Ferrous sulphate*: tetracycline decreases the absorption of ferrous sulphate

Route of administration
- Oral, topical, IM, IV

Note
- Most Gram positive and several Gram negative bacteria are now resistant to tetracycline (resistance is mediated by plasmids).
- Tetracycline chelates calcium and is therefore deposited in growing bones and teeth. This leads to discoloration of teeth and should therefore not be given to children under 8 years of age or to lactating or pregnant women.
- Tetracycline should not be taken with food or milk (impaired absorption).
- Doxycycline is preferred to tetracycline as it does not affect renal function.

Related drugs
- Doxycycline, oxytetracycline

Trimethoprim

Class: Antifolate antibiotic

Indications
- Urinary tract infection (caused by, for example, *Escherichia coli*, *Proteus mirabilis*)
- Prostatitis

Mechanism of action
- Trimethoprim reduces bacterial production of folate by inhibiting the bacterial enzyme dihydrofolate reductase (trimethoprim has a 50 000 times greater affinity for bacterial dihydrofolate reductase than for the human enzyme).
- Trimethoprim is bacteriostatic, as folate is an essential cofactor in DNA synthesis.

Adverse effects
- *Rare*: bone marrow suppression, nausea, vomiting, rash, toxic epidermal necrolysis

Contraindications
- Pregnancy (due to teratogenic effects)
- Severe renal impairment
- Blood disorders (e.g. anaemia, thrombocytopenia)

Interactions
- *Cyclosporin*: concomitant use of cyclosporin and trimethoprim increases the risk of nephrotoxicity
- *Pyrimethamine*: concomitant use of pyrimethamine and trimethoprim can enhance the antifolate effect

Route of administration
- Oral, IV

Note
- Resistance to trimethoprim is common.
- Folate deficiency can be avoided by giving folinic acid.
- Trimethoprim can be used in combination with a sulphonamide (sulphamethoxazole) as co-trimoxazole, which is bactericidal. This combination produces synergistic activity (especially effective for *Pneumocystis carinii* infections).

Zidovudine

Class: Nucleoside reverse transcriptase inhibitor

Indications
- Part of combination therapy for HIV infection
- Prevention of HIV transmission from mother to fetus

Mechanism of action
- Zidovudine is a nucleoside analogue. It is phosphorylated inside cells to form zidovudine triphosphate, which is a competitive inhibitor of viral reverse transcriptase. Zidovudine triphosphate is also incorporated into proviral DNA, thus terminating DNA chain elongation.
- Zidovudine does not eradicate HIV from the body.

Adverse effects
- *Common*: anaemia, neutropenia, headache, insomnia, nausea, abdominal pain
- *Rare*: convulsions, myalgia, myopathy

Contraindications
- Low neutrophil count
- Severe anaemia
- Breast feeding

Interactions
- *Fluconazole*: fluconazole increases the risk of zidovudine toxicity by raising its plasma concentration
- ***Ganciclovir***: ganciclovir causes severe myelosuppression with zidovudine
- *Probenecid*: probenecid increases the risk of zidovudine toxicity by raising its plasma concentration

Route of administration
- Oral, IV infusion

Note
- Resistance to zidovudine develops as a result of mutations in viral reverse transcriptase. Combined therapy (two nucleoside reverse transcriptase inhibitors + *either* a non-nucleoside reverse transcriptase inhibitor *or* a protease inhibitor) is given in order to prevent emergence of resistant strains.
- Therapy is guided by HIV viral load and CD4 count.
- Blood transfusions are frequently required as zidovudine causes anaemia.

Related drugs
- Didanosine, lamivudine, stavudine, zalcitabine

IMMUNIZATION

RECOMMENDED IMMUNIZATION PROGRAMME IN THE UK

Vaccine	Age
Hepatitis B (for infants at risk)	Birth, 1 month and 6 months
DTP, polio, Hib	2, 3 and 4 months
MMR	12 months
DT, polio, MMR	3–5 years (pre-school booster)
BCG	10–14 years (given at birth if at risk)
DT (low dose), polio	13–18 years (school leavers)

• If the immunization course is interrupted, there is no need to restart the entire course

CONTRAINDICATIONS TO ALL VACCINES
• Acute febrile illness
• Severe reaction to a previous dose

CONTRAINDICATIONS TO LIVE VACCINES (BCG, MMR, POLIO)
• Immunocompromised patients
• Pregnancy
• Patients with HIV/AIDS (omit BCG, but can receive MMR and polio)
• High dose corticosteroids (wait for 3 months after stopping the treatment)
• Chemo/radiotherapy (wait for 6 months after stopping the treatment)
• Another live vaccine within the past 3 weeks
• Acute febrile illness
• Severe reaction to a previous dose

BCG vaccine (Bacillus Calmette–Guérin)

Class: Live attenuated vaccine

Indications
- Prophylaxis against tuberculosis

Mechanism of action
- BCG vaccine contains a live attenuated strain derived from *Mycobacterium bovis*. This induces a hypersensitivity reaction and thereby stimulates cell-mediated immunity against *Mycobacterium tuberculosis*.

Adverse effects
- *Common*: ulcer at injection site
- *Rare*: axillary lymphadenopathy, tuberculosis (in the immunocompromised)

Contraindications
- The first 3 weeks following another live vaccine
- Pregnancy
- Acute febrile illness
- Immunocompromised patients (e.g. steroid therapy, immunosuppressive drugs, HIV, malignancy)

Interactions
- None

Route of administration
- Intradermal injection

Note
- BCG vaccine should only be given if the Heaf test or Mantoux test is negative.
- An ulcer usually appears at the site of injection 2–3 weeks after the vaccination. This normally heals within 6–12 weeks.
- It is standard practice to give the vaccine into the left arm so that BCG status can be easily checked, as the injection leaves a characteristic scar for life.

Diphtheria vaccine

Class: Toxoid vaccine

Indications
- Prophylaxis against diphtheria

Mechanism of action
- Diphtheria vaccine contains inactivated diphtheria toxin (toxoid), which stimulates production of antibodies. These provide immunity against *Corynebacterium diphtheriae*.

Adverse effects
- *Common*: pain and swelling at the injection site
- *Rare*: fever

Contraindications
- Acute febrile illness
- Severe reaction to a previous dose

Interactions
- None

Route of administration
- IM, deep subcutaneous

Note
- The vaccine is given to children as part of the triple vaccine (DTP vaccine). It is also given to travellers going to areas where diphtheria is prevalent.
- Adults and children over 10 years of age who require a primary dose or a booster should be given the low dose vaccine.
- Diphtheria should be treated with antitoxin and an antibiotic (e.g. benzylpenicillin).

Hepatitis B vaccine

Class: Subunit vaccine

Indications
- Prophylaxis against hepatitis B

Mechanism of action
- The vaccine contains hepatitis B surface antigen (HBsAg), which is prepared in yeast by recombinant DNA technology. It stimulates production of anti-HBsAg antibodies, which confers protective immunity.

Adverse effects
- *Common*: discomfort at the injection site
- *Rare*: anaphylaxis

Contraindications
- Acute febrile illness
- Severe reaction to a previous dose

Interactions
- None

Route of administration
- IM (deltoid muscle, not gluteal), subcutaneous (to avoid bleeding in haemophilia patients)

Note
- Hepatitis B vaccine should be given to those at high risk (e.g. health care workers, haemophiliacs, babies born to infected mothers).
- A post-vaccination period of up to 6 months is required in order to achieve a protective level of antibodies. Boosters every 5 years are recommended.
- Following a single episode of exposure to hepatitis B virus (e.g. contact with infected blood), injection of hepatitis B-specific immunoglobulin should be given as soon as possible. This confers a significant level of protection against the disease.

Hib vaccine

Class: Inactivated vaccine

Indications
- Prophylaxis against *Haemophilus influenzae* type b (Hib) infections

Mechanism of action
- Hib vaccine contains a capsular polysaccharide obtained from *Haemophilus influenzae* type b, which has been conjugated to a protein carrier (this enhances immunogenicity).
- Administration stimulates an antibody response.

Adverse effects
- *Common*: fever, headache, anorexia, diarrhoea, vomiting
- *Rare*: convulsions, erythema multiforme

Contraindications
- Acute febrile illness
- Severe reaction to a previous dose

Interactions
- None

Route of administration
- IM, deep subcutaneous

Note
- The main reason for vaccination is to prevent epiglottitis and meningitis.
- Hib vaccine is not usually required for children over 4 years of age because the risk of infection with *Haemophilus influenzae* type b falls rapidly after this age. Exceptions to this rule are patients with sickle-cell disease, asplenic patients and those on treatment for malignancy.

MMR vaccine

Class: Live combined vaccine

Indications
- Prophylaxis against mumps, measles and rubella (MMR)

Mechanism of action
- MMR vaccine contains live attenuated strains of mumps, measles and rubella viruses.
- It provides active immunity by causing the production of antibodies to these organisms.

Adverse effects
- *Common*: fever, malaise, rash
- *Rare*: parotid swelling

Contraindications
- Immunocompromised children
- Pregnancy
- The first 3 weeks following another live vaccine
- Allergy to neomycin or kanamycin (MMR vaccine contains traces of both)
- Acute febrile illness
- Severe reaction to a previous dose

Interactions
- None

Route of administration
- IM, deep subcutaneous

Note
- Women should avoid pregnancy for 1 month following MMR vaccination.
- MMR vaccine does not provide effective protection following exposure to mumps or rubella virus because the antibody response to these components of the vaccine is too slow.
- Adverse effects commonly occur following the first dose and much less so following the second dose of MMR vaccine.
- The link between MMR vaccine and both autism and inflammatory bowel disease has been disproved.

Pertussis vaccine

Class: Inactivated vaccine

Indications
- Prophylaxis of whooping cough

Mechanism of action
- Pertussis vaccine contains killed *Bordetella pertussis* organism. The vaccine induces active immunity by formation of antibodies against *Bordetella pertussis*, thus protecting against whooping cough.

Adverse effects
- *Common*: fever, pain and redness at the injection site
- *Rare*: encephalopathy, convulsions, oedema and induration of the limb into which the injection was given

Contraindications
- Acute febrile illness
- Severe reaction to a previous dose

Interactions
- None

Route of administration
- IM, deep subcutaneous

Note
- Acellular pertussis vaccine is given to those who have had a serious reaction to a previous dose. It is only available on a named patient basis.
- Parents are frequently concerned about pertussis vaccine, as an association with brain damage has been reported. Parents should be informed that the risk of brain damage due to whooping cough is far greater than the risk associated with the vaccine.

Polio vaccine

Class: Live-attenuated or inactivated vaccine

Indications
  • Prophylaxis against poliomyelitis
Mechanism of action
  • The oral polio vaccine contains live attenuated strains of polioviruses. It induces active immunity by formation of IgG and IgA antibodies thereby conferring protection against CNS and GI infections.
  • The inactivated subcutaneous vaccine induces the formation of IgG antibodies only.
Adverse effects
  • *Rare*: paralysis with oral vaccine (less than 1 in 2 million doses)
Contraindications
  • Sabin vaccine (oral):
    • Vomiting and diarrhoea
    • Immunosuppression
    • Pregnancy
    • Severe reaction to a previous dose
    • Malignancy
Interactions
  • None
Route of administration
  • Salk vaccine: subcutaneous
  • Sabin vaccine: oral
Note
  • There are two types of polio vaccine: Sabin oral vaccine (live) and Salk subcutaneous vaccine (inactivated).
  • Salk vaccine is used only if Sabin vaccine is contraindicated due to immunosuppression.
  • Poliomyelitis is endemic in developing countries and therefore unimmunized travellers to countries other than New Zealand, Australia, North America or Northern or Western Europe should be vaccinated (unless previously vaccinated).
  • Orally vaccinated children are usually infectious to others for about 6 weeks due to shedding of the virus in the faeces.

Tetanus vaccine

Class: Toxoid vaccine

Indications
- Prophylaxis against tetanus

Mechanism of action
- Tetanus vaccine contains inactivated tetanus toxin (toxoid) which stimulates the immune system to produce antibodies thus inducing active immunity.

Adverse effects
- *Common*: pain and swelling at the site of injection
- *Rare*: fever

Contraindications
- Acute febrile illness
- Severe reaction to a previous dose

Interactions
- None

Route of administration
- IM

Note
- A full course of tetanus immunization should be given to both non-immunized individuals and to those with unknown immunization status following a penetrating injury or burns (three vaccines given monthly and a booster every 10 years).
- Following an injury in a previously immunized individual, a booster should be given only if more than 10 years have elapsed since the last dose.

OBSTETRICS AND GYNAECOLOGY

This chapter provides a description of the treatments and procedures commonly encountered in obstetrics and gynaecology. We have included an overview of HRT and contraception. This is followed by a detailed account of relevant drugs.

INDUCTION OF LABOUR
- Assess the state of the cervix prior to induction
- Unripe cervix must be ripened with vaginal prostaglandins (e.g. PGE_2)
- If this fails consider caesarean section
- Once the cervix is ripe, rupture the membranes
- Monitor fetal heart
- If necessary, give IV oxytocin until effective uterine contractions are present (sometimes given until delivery)
- Manage as high-risk labour
- A combination of ergometrine and oxytocin is used to accelerate the 3rd stage of labour and reduce the risk of postpartum haemorrhage

PRE-ECLAMPSIA
- The objective of treatment is to prevent eclampsia (maternal convulsions during pregnancy)
- Admit if blood pressure is greater than 140/90 mmHg with proteinuria and oedema
- Advise bed rest
- Monitor blood pressure 2–4 hourly, urine protein, plasma urate, platelet count and the fetus (CTG)
- Control blood pressure with antihypertensives:
IV hydralazine or IV labetolol or oral nifedipine

HYPERTENSION IN PREGNANCY
- Admit if blood pressure exceeds 160/100 mmHg in a known hypertensive
- Advise bed rest
- Monitor blood pressure 2–4 hourly, urine protein, plasma urate, platelet count and the fetus (CTG)
- If high blood pressure persists, treat with antihypertensives (see below)
- If high blood pressure persists with proteinuria, treat as for pre-eclampsia

Pharmacological treatment
- Treat if blood pressure reaches 160/105 mmHg
- Drugs that are commonly used:
  1 Oral methyldopa

2 Oral β blocker (e.g. atenolol)
3 Oral nifedipine

ECLAMPSIA
• Give IV magnesium sulphate
• Delivery is the only cure
• Test patellar reflexes regularly after giving magnesium sulphate (loss of reflexes is an early sign of toxicity)
• The mother must be monitored after delivery, as eclampsia can occur postpartum (especially within the first 48 hours)

MENORRHAGIA
• Treat any underlying cause (e.g. pelvic pathology, clotting disorder, medical disorders)
• In most cases no cause is found (termed dysfunctional uterine bleeding) and treatment is mainly symptomatic:
  1 Medical treatment
     • To decrease blood loss: antifibrinolytics (e.g. tranexamic acid), NSAIDs (e.g. mefenamic acid) or systemic progestogens
     • To restore a regular cycle: COC pill
  2 Progesterone loaded IUCD
  3 Surgical treatment
     • Endometrial resection or ablation
     • Myomectomy for fibroids (only performed if further pregnancies are desired, as the complication rate is greater than for hysterectomy)
     • Hysterectomy in severe cases

CONTRACEPTION
• 90% of fertile young females who have regular unprotected intercourse become pregnant within 1 year

Methods of contraception
1 Natural methods: rhythm method, coitus interruptus
2 Barrier methods: male or female condom, diaphragm, cap
3 IUCD
4 Hormonal: COC pill, progestogen-only pill (POP), depot injection, subcutaneous implant
5 Sterilization: vasectomy in males, laparoscopic occlusion of the Fallopian tubes in females

Post-coital contraception
• 'Morning-after pill' (contains levonorgestrel and ethinyloestradiol)—give two tablets within 72 hours following sexual intercourse, followed by two more tablets 12 hours later
• Alternatively, an IUCD can be placed within 5 days following unprotected intercourse

HORMONE REPLACEMENT THERAPY
The climacteric/menopause
• Begins between the ages of 45 and 55 years, when the female menstrual periods cease
• Symptoms of the menopause are due to lack of oestrogens

Types of HRT
1 In women with a uterus: give preparations containing oestrogen and a progestogen
2 In women without a uterus: give preparations containing oestrogen only

Benefits of HRT
1 Symptomatic relief of postmenopausal symptoms (e.g. sweating, flushing, atrophic vaginitis, irritability)
2 Prevention of menopause-associated disease processes (e.g. CHD, stroke, osteoporosis, ovarian cancer, Alzheimer's disease)
3 A progestogen is added to HRT in order to prevent cystic hyperplasia and oestrogen-related cancer of the endometrium

Disadvantages of HRT
1 Adverse effects of oestrogen and progestogen
2 Possible increased risk of breast cancer and endometrial cancer

Note
• HRT can be given orally or as a patch, gel or subcutaneous implant.
• Long term use of HRT may be linked to breast cancer, hence regular mammograms are recommended.

Ergometrine

Class: Ergot alkaloid

Indications
- Routine management of the 3rd stage of labour
- Prevention and treatment of postpartum haemorrhage

Mechanism of action
- Exact mechanism is not fully understood.
- It may act at α adrenoceptors, prostaglandin and serotonin receptors.
- Ergometrine causes uterine contractions and has some degree of vasoconstrictor action.

Adverse effects
- *Common*: nausea, vomiting, abdominal pain, hypertension

Contraindications
- Induction of labour
- 1st and 2nd stages of labour
- Eclampsia
- Hypertension
- Peripheral vascular disease (due to vasoconstrictor action)
- Severe cardiac impairment
- Severe hepatic impairment
- Severe renal impairment

Interactions
- None

Route of administration
- Oral, IM, IV (in emergencies)

Note
- Ergometrine is often given together with oxytocin in the 3rd stage of labour or in postpartum haemorrhage. These two drugs, when combined, are more effective than either one of them alone.
- Due to its vasoconstrictor action, ergometrine may cause spasm of the coronary arteries, resulting in anginal pain.

Oestrogens

Class: Sex hormones

Indications
- Combined oral contraceptive pill (COC pill)
- Hormone replacement therapy
- Atrophic vaginitis (topical use)

Mechanism of action
- In HRT, replacing the deficient oestrogen alleviates menopausal symptoms.
- Given as the COC pill, oestrogens inhibit the release of FSH from the anterior pituitary by negative feedback. This prevents maturation of the Graafian follicle in the ovary.

Adverse effects
- *Common*: fluid retention, hypertension, loss of libido, nausea, vomiting, breast tenderness, weight gain, acne, mood swings, worsened migraine
- *Rare*: thromboembolic events, headache, depression, slightly increased risk of breast cancer, slightly increased risk of endometrial cancer (only if given alone without a progestogen), hepatic tumours

Contraindications
- Pregnancy
- Breast feeding
- Previous thromboembolic events (PE, DVT)
- Hepatic disease (oestrogens are metabolized by the liver)
- Oestrogen-dependent tumours (e.g. endometrial cancer)
- Focal migraine

Interactions
- ***Broad-spectrum antibiotics***: these may decrease the effects of oestrogens by impairing the gut flora responsible for recycling ethinyloestradiol in the large bowel
- ***Carbamazepine***: carbamazepine increases the metabolism of oestrogens, thereby decreasing their effect
- ***Phenytoin, rifampicin***: these drugs decrease the plasma concentration of oestrogens
- ***Warfarin***: oestrogens reduce the anticoagulant effect of warfarin

Route of administration
- Oral, transdermal patch (lasts about 24 hours), subcutaneous implant (lasts 4–8 months), vaginal cream, pessary

Note
- Blood pressure should be checked regularly with prolonged use (risk of hypertension).
- The COC pill failure rate is 5 pregnancies per 1000 women years of administration.
- The COC pill (containing both an oestrogen and a progestogen) protects against endometrial and ovarian cancer.
- Oestrogens may need to be discontinued several weeks prior to surgery, as they predispose to thromboembolic events.

Oxytocin

Class: Oxytocic agent

Indications
- Induction of labour
- Management of the 3rd stage of labour
- To cause uterine contraction after Caesarean section
- Prevention and treatment of postpartum haemorrhage
- Spontaneous abortion

Mechanism of action
- Oxytocin produces contractions of the fundus in the pregnant uterus by acting on local oxytocin receptors.
- It also enhances uterine contractions by increasing the production of prostaglandins in the myometrium.

Adverse effects
- *Common*: uterine spasm, nausea, vomiting
- *Rare*: fluid and electrolyte disturbance, hypotension, tachycardia, dysrhythmias

Contraindications
- Mechanical obstruction in pregnancy and any other condition where vaginal delivery is not advisable
- Predisposition to uterine rupture
- Fetal distress

Interactions
- No serious interactions

Route of administration
- IV

Note
- Oxytocin should be discontinued in cases of uterine hyperactivity or fetal distress.
- Careful monitoring of fetal heart rate and uterine contractions is required when oxytocin is used in labour.
- Oxytocin is often given together with ergometrine in the 3rd stage of labour or in postpartum haemorrhage. These two drugs, when combined, are more effective than either one of them alone.

Progestogens

Class: Sex hormones

Indications
- Contraception
- Part of HRT
- Menstrual disorders (e.g. dysmenorrhoea, menorrhagia)
- Endometriosis
- Neoplastic disease (endometrial cancer, renal cell carcinoma, 2nd or 3rd line therapy in the treatment of breast cancer)

Mechanism of action
- The main contraceptive effect of progestogens is due to their action on cervical mucus which is rendered impenetrable to sperm. Progestogens also prevent implantation of the fertilized ovum.
- Progestogens suppress the secretion of gonadotrophins from the anterior pituitary by negative feedback, thus inhibiting ovulation in about 40% of females.
- In endometriosis, progestogens are used to inhibit menstruation, thus producing regression of smaller lesions.

Adverse effects
- *Common*: menstrual irregularities, breast tenderness, weight gain, acne, bloating, nausea, vomiting, depression
- *Rare*: cholestatic jaundice

Contraindications
- Pregnancy
- Severe hypertension
- Unexplained vaginal bleeding
- Hepatic impairment

Interactions
- *Rifamycins*: reduced contraceptive effect
- *Cyclosporin*: progestogens increase the plasma concentration of cyclosporin

Route of administration
- Oral, IM, subdermal implant, IUCD, vaginal gel, rectal

Note
- Progestogens are divided into two main classes: progesterone with its analogues (hydroxyprogesterone, dydrogesterone, medroxyprogesterone) and testosterone analogues (norgestrel, norethisterone). Gestodene, desogestrel and norgestimate are derivatives of norgestrel.
- The progestogen-only pill (POP) is given when combined oral contraceptives are contraindicated (e.g. history of thromboembolic disease). However, the POP has a slightly higher failure rate than the combined pill.
- The POP must be taken at the same time each day. The contraceptive effect is inadequate if administration is delayed by more than 3 hours. In this case the pill should be continued as normal, but a different method of contraception (e.g. condom) should be used for a period of 1 week.

ENDOCRINE SYSTEM

This chapter provides an account of the management of diabetes mellitus and thyroid disorders followed by a detailed account of drugs used in endocrinology.

DIABETES MELLITUS
Diabetes mellitus type I
- Insulin is always required (amount is tailored to the individual)
- Regular monitoring of blood glucose is required
- Compliance is essential to maintain optimal glucose levels and thus minimize the risk of long term complications (e.g. retinopathy, peripheral neuropathy, nephropathy)

Diabetes mellitus type II
- Recommend diet therapy (reduce fat intake, increase intake of complex carbohydrates such as pasta and potatoes) and physical exercise
- Metformin is the treatment of choice in patients not responding to diet (unless BMI < 20 kg/m^2, in which case a sulphonylurea is the 1st choice)
- Give insulin if HbA1c remains unacceptably high (> 7–8%)

COMPLICATIONS OF DIABETES MELLITUS
Hypoglycaemia
- Give oral glucose
- If no improvement give 50 mL of 50% dextrose IV or glucagon IM

Ketoacidosis
- Give IV fluids
- Give insulin until glucose levels are within normal range and anion gap or arterial pH have normalized
- Continue with subcutaneous insulin bolus when the patient starts eating
- Monitor plasma potassium (administer potassium when it reaches the normal range in order to prevent insulin-induced hypokalaemia)
- Insert nasogastric tube in comatose patients to prevent aspiration pneumonia
- Investigate the cause

Hyperglycaemic hyperosmotic non-ketotic coma
- Give IV fluids (use 0.45% saline if plasma Na$^+$ > 150 mmol/L)
- Give heparin (to prevent deep venous thrombosis)
- Give insulin until glucose levels are within the normal range

- Monitor plasma potassium (administer potassium if levels fall)
- Investigate the cause

HYPOTHYROIDISM
- Thyroxine replacement for life
- Monitor thyroid function at regular intervals to ensure TSH is within the normal range

HYPERTHYROIDISM
- Control symptoms of hyperthyroidism with a β blocker (e.g. propranolol)
- Give an antithyroid agent (e.g. carbimazole)
- If hyperthyroidism persists, oral radioactive iodide solution can be given
- Consider subtotal thyroidectomy if the above measures fail
- In thyrotoxic crisis give IV fluids, IV propranolol, IV hydrocortisone, oral iodine and oral carbimazole

Calcitonin

Class: Hormone

Indications
- Paget's disease of the bone
- Hypercalcaemia
- Bone pain in malignancy
- Osteoporosis (menopausal and steroid-induced)

Mechanism of action
- Calcitonin lowers serum calcium.
- Calcitonin decreases bone resorption by inhibiting the activity of osteoclasts and by reducing their number.
- It also increases renal calcium excretion.

Adverse effects
- *Common*: nausea, vomiting, flushing
- *Rare*: tingling in the hand, inflammation at the injection site, unpleasant taste in the mouth

Contraindications
- Breast feeding

Interactions
- None

Route of administration
- IV infusion, IM, subcutaneous

Note
- Two types of calcitonin preparations are available: porcine (natural) and salcatonin (synthetic). Both are immunogenic (antibodies can be made against them), but salcatonin is less so and is thus more suitable in long term therapy.
- Calcium supplements should be given in conjunction with calcitonin.
- If HRT is not tolerated or is inappropriate, a combination of calcitonin, bisphosphonate and calcium supplements can be used to treat osteoporosis.
- In Paget's disease of the bone, calcitonin decreases pain and may prevent neurological complications.

Carbimazole

Class: Antithyroid drug

Indications
- Hyperthyroidism

Mechanism of action
- Carbimazole decreases the production of thyroid hormones T3 (tri-iodothyronine) and T4 (thyroxine) in the thyroid.
- It has several actions. The main ones are iodine trapping and inhibition of the enzyme thyroid peroxidase, which is necessary for thyroid hormone synthesis.

Adverse effects
- *Common*: GI disturbance, headache, skin rash, pruritus, joint pain
- *Rare*: agranulocytosis, jaundice, alopecia

Contraindications
- None
- Caution:
  - Breast feeding
  - Pregnancy (low doses should be used as carbimazole in high dose crosses the placenta and can cause neonatal hypothyroidism or goitre)

Interactions
- None

Route of administration
- Oral

Note
- Treatment of Graves' disease should continue for at least 1 year. Recurrence of hyperthyroidism occurs in more than half of the patients, but can be treated with another course of carbimazole.
- All patients must be advised to seek medical help if they develop signs of bone marrow suppression (e.g. sore throat, mouth ulcers). If a low neutrophil count is confirmed, treatment must be discontinued. If not, treatment should be continued.
- Carbimazole can be replaced with propylthiouracil if rash and itching cannot be tolerated.
- Regular monitoring of thyroid function is essential.

Related drugs
- Propylthiouracil

Desmopressin

Class: Synthetic ADH analogue

Indications
- Treatment and diagnosis of pituitary diabetes insipidus
- Persistent enuresis
- Haemophilia
- Postoperative polyuria/polydipsia

Mechanism of action
- Desmopressin mimics the action of ADH.
- It selectively activates V_2 receptors in renal tubular cells. This causes increased reabsorption of water and decreased excretion of sodium and water, thus controlling polyuria and polydipsia.
- In haemophilia, desmopressin increases the plasma concentration of factor VIII.

Adverse effects
- *Common*: dilutional hyponatraemia, fluid retention
- *Rare*: nausea, vomiting, abdominal cramps

Contraindications
- Heart failure

Interactions
- No serious interactions

Route of administration
- Oral, intranasal, IM, IV, subcutaneous

Note
- Desmopressin is used in the water deprivation test to differentiate between pituitary and nephrogenic diabetes insipidus.
- Unlike vasopressin, desmopressin has no vasoconstrictor effect. Therefore desmopressin cannot be used in the treatment of bleeding oesophageal varices.
- To avoid water intoxication, doses should be adjusted to allow some diuresis.

Related drugs
- Felypressin, lypressin, terlipressin, vasopressin (ADH)

Gliclazide

Class: Sulphonylurea

Indications
- Type II diabetes mellitus (only in the presence of some pancreatic β-cell activity as gliclazide requires the presence of endogenous insulin)

Mechanism of action
- Gliclazide stimulates insulin production by binding to sulphonylurea receptors and blocking ATP-dependent potassium channels in pancreatic β cells. This causes depolarization and insulin release.
- Gliclazide also inhibits gluconeogenesis.

Adverse effects
- *Common*: hypoglycaemia, weight gain
- *Rare*: headache, rash, GI disturbance, bone marrow suppression

Contraindications
- Ketoacidosis
- Pregnancy
- Breast feeding
- Caution:
  - The elderly and patients with hepatic or renal impairment are very susceptible to hypoglycaemia

Interactions
- *Chloramphenicol, cotrimoxazole and sulphonamides*: these enhance the hypoglycaemic effect of gliclazide
- *Fluconazole*: fluconazole increases the plasma concentration of gliclazide

Route of administration
- Oral

Note
- Gliclazide is used in thin patients with type II diabetes mellitus not responding to diet alone.
- Gliclazide is often combined with metformin in those who cannot achieve adequate glycaemic control with either of these two drugs alone.
- As sulphonylureas do not provide adequate glycaemic control during surgery and illness (e.g. infection, MI, trauma), they are usually temporarily substituted with insulin for these events.

Related drugs
- Chlorpropamide (long acting, increased risk of adverse effects), glibenclamide, glimepiride, glipizide, tolazamide, tolbutamide

Insulin

Class: Peptide hormone

Indications
- Diabetes mellitus type I
- Diabetes mellitus type II
- Ketoacidosis
- Hyperglycaemic hyperosmotic non-ketotic coma
- Emergency treatment of hyperkalaemia (IV glucose must be coadministered)

Mechanism of action
- Insulin lowers plasma glucose concentration through the following actions:
  1 it stimulates glucose transport into fat and muscle cells;
  2 it stimulates glycogen synthesis; and
  3 it inhibits gluconeogenesis and lipolysis.

Adverse effects
- *Common*: hypoglycaemia, weight gain
- *Rare*: fat hypertrophy at the injection site (sites should be rotated)

Contraindications
- None
- Caution:
  - Renal impairment (may require lower doses)

Interactions
- *β blockers*: β blockers mask the warning signs of hypoglycaemia which are predominantly mediated by the sympathetic nervous system

Route of administration
- Subcutaneous, IM, IV infusion

Note
- There are three different types of insulin preparations:
  1 Short-acting preparations (soluble insulin, insulin lispro)—duration of action up to 7 hours.
  2 Intermediate-acting preparations (e.g. insulin zinc suspension, isophane insulin)—duration of action 14–22 hours.
  3 Long-acting preparations (e.g. crystalline insulin zinc suspension)—duration of action 36 hours.
- Stress, infection, trauma and pregnancy can increase insulin requirements.
- Insulin promotes the influx of potassium as well as glucose into cells. As a consequence the plasma potassium concentration can drop to dangerously low levels, particularly during insulin treatment of ketoacidosis. In this situation potassium must be replaced intravenously.

Metformin

Class: Biguanide

Indications
- Type II diabetes mellitus

Mechanism of action
- The exact mechanism is not fully understood.
- Metformin requires the presence of insulin, as it is principally an insulin-sensitizing agent.
- Metformin does not influence insulin release. It increases peripheral glucose utilization and decreases gluconeogenesis, possibly through its action on membrane phospholipids.
- It also inhibits glucose absorption from the intestinal lumen.

Adverse effects
- *Common*: anorexia, nausea, vomiting, diarrhoea
- *Rare*: lactic acidosis (especially in renal impairment)

Contraindications
- Pregnancy
- Breast feeding
- *Note*: The following conditions predispose to lactic acidosis and are therefore contraindicated:
  - Hepatic impairment
  - Renal impairment
  - Severe heart failure
  - Severe infection
  - Severe dehydration

Interactions
- *Alcohol*: excessive alcohol intake with metformin can predispose to lactic acidosis
- *Corticosteroids*: corticosteroids antagonize the hypoglycaemic effect of metformin

Route of administration
- Oral

Note
- Metformin does not cause hypoglycaemia.
- It is used in type II diabetes mellitus patients who do not respond to diet control.
- Metformin reduces appetite, thus encouraging weight loss. It is therefore the treatment of choice in obese diabetics.

Thyroxine sodium

Class: Thyroid hormone

Indications
- Hypothyroidism

Mechanism of action
- Thyroxine sodium mimics endogenous thyroxine, thus increasing oxygen consumption of metabolically active tissues.

Adverse effects
- *Rare*: cardiac dysrhythmias, tachycardia, myocardial infarction, anginal pain, restlessness, sweating, weight loss (all with excessive doses)

Contraindications
- None

Interactions
- *Warfarin*: thyroxine increases the effect of warfarin

Route of administration
- Oral

Note
- Plasma thyroid-stimulating hormone (TSH) levels should be monitored to assess treatment. TSH levels return to normal 6 weeks after optimum thyroxine levels are achieved.
- Thyroxine should be introduced gradually in patients with ischaemic heart disease, as thyroxine can cause excessive cardiac stimulation (consider a pretherapy ECG).

Related drugs
- Liothyronine sodium (faster acting than thyroxine sodium)

GENERAL ANAESTHESIA

General anaesthetic agents are employed as an adjunct to surgical procedures. They achieve a state of complete and reversible loss of consciousness in which the patient is unaware of and unresponsive to painful stimuli.

Unlike local anaesthetics, general anaesthetics are given systemically. They produce their effects by acting on the CNS, whilst maintaining the functioning of other body systems such as the cardiovascular and respiratory systems.

Agents used in general anaesthesia are manifold and can be divided into the following categories.

Premedication (given before induction of general anaesthesia)
• Benzodiazepines to reduce anxiety
• Antimuscarinics (e.g. hyoscine, atropine) to reduce secretions and vagal reflexes

Anaesthetic agents
• Induction of general anaesthesia by IV agents:
    1 Non-barbiturates (e.g. propofol, ketamine, etomidate)
    2 Barbiturates (thiopentone, methohexitone)
• Maintenance of anaesthesia by inhalational agents (e.g. isoflurane, sevoflurane)

Muscle relaxation
• Depolarizing (e.g. suxamethonium) and non-depolarizing (e.g. atracurium) muscle relaxants are used to facilitate surgery
• After surgery the effects of non-depolarizing muscle relaxants are reversed by anticholinesterase drugs (e.g. neostigmine)

Analgesia (used perioperatively)
• Opioids in conjunction with an anti-emetic
• NSAIDs (e.g. ibuprofen, diclofenac)
• Local anaesthetics (lidocaine, bupivacaine)
• Paracetamol

LOCAL ANAESTHESIA

Local anaesthetics are the method of choice for many minor surgical procedures. They are especially useful in patients suffering from severe cardio-respiratory disease who are more susceptible to the risks of general anaesthetics.

Agents used to induce local anaesthesia (e.g. lidocaine) act by causing a local nerve conduction block.

Atracurium

Class: Non-depolarizing muscle relaxant

Indications
- To achieve muscle relaxation in general anaesthesia
- Long term mechanical ventilation in ITU

Mechanism of action
- Atracurium competitively binds to nicotinic acetylcholine receptors at motor end-plates, thus causing paralysis of skeletal muscle.

Adverse effects
- *Common*: skin rash, flushing, hypotension (all associated with histamine release)
- *Rare*: anaphylactoid reactions, bronchospasm

Contraindications
- Asthma

Interactions
- *Aminoglycosides*: aminoglycosides enhance the effects of atracurium
- *Clindamycin*: clindamycin enhances the effects of atracurium

Route of administration
- IV

Note
- The action of atracurium is reversible with an anticholinesterase agent (e.g. neostigmine).
- Atracurium has an intermediate duration of action (30–45 min).
- Atracurium is unique as it undergoes inactivation in the plasma and thus can be used in patients with hepatic or renal impairment.
- Non-depolarizing muscle relaxants of short/intermediate duration of action (e.g. atracurium, vecuronium) are more widely used than those of long duration of action (e.g. pancuronium).

Related drugs
- Cisatracurium, mivacurium, pancuronium, rocuronium, vecuronium

Isoflurane

Class: Inhalational anaesthetic agent

Indications
- Maintenance of anaesthesia

Mechanism of action
- The exact mechanism is not fully understood.
- Most theories infer that general anaesthetic agents act on the cell membrane.
- Three important theories have been put forward:
  1 Lipid theory—anaesthetics change the lipid component of cell membranes and thus alter transmembrane ion movements to produce anaesthesia.
  2 Protein theory—anaesthetics bind to proteins and reversibly change their structure to induce anaesthesia.
  3 Hydrate theory—anaesthetics produce crystals within cell membranes by freezing the water component of the membrane, thus producing anaesthesia.

Adverse effects
- *Common*: coughing and breathholding on induction due to pungent odour (hence not used for induction), respiratory depression, hypotension, tachycardia
- *Rare*: hepatotoxicity

Contraindications
- Hypersensitivity (rare but known)
- Malignant hyperpyrexia

Interactions
- *Antihypertensives*: antihypertensives enhance the hypotensive effect of isoflurane

Route of administration
- Inhalation

Note
- Isoflurane is commonly used as it has a much lower incidence of hepatotoxicity than halothane or enflurane.
- Isoflurane has little effect on the heart, unlike halothane and enflurane.

Related drugs
- Desflurane, enflurane, halothane, sevoflurane

Lidocaine (lignocaine)

Class: Local anaesthetic, class I anti-arrhythmic agent

Indications
- Local anaesthesia
- Ventricular dysrhythmias (especially following myocardial infarction)

Mechanism of action
- Lidocaine blocks fast sodium channels in nerve axons. This inhibits the generation of action potentials, thus causing a reversible nerve conduction block.
- Lidocaine suppresses premature ventricular beats and ventricular tachycardia by slowing the conduction velocity along the Purkinje fibres and ventricular muscle. This action is achieved by blockade of fast sodium channels.

Adverse effects
- *Common*: nausea, vomiting, drowsiness, dizziness
- *Rare*: bradycardia, hypotension, cardiac arrest, convulsions, confusion, coma

Contraindications
- All degrees of AV node block
- Myocardial depression
- Severe heart failure
- SA node disorders
- Hypovolaemia
- Porphyria

Interactions
- *β blockers*: β blockers increase the risk of lidocaine toxicity (dizziness, seizures)
- *Cimetidine*: cimetidine increases the risk of lidocaine toxicity by inhibiting its metabolism

Route of administration
- IV (dysrhythmias only); subdural, epidural; intradermal or subcutaneous injection at a desired site; topical application to mucous membranes and skin

Note
- Extreme care must be taken to avoid accidental intravenous injection during administration of local anaesthesia.
- Solutions containing lidocaine and epinephrine must not be used in ring block anaesthesia (e.g. fingers, toes, penis) as this may cause ischaemic necrosis. Instead, solutions containing only lidocaine should be used.
- Lidocaine must not be injected into inflamed or infected tissue as this may cause systemic effects (due to rapid absorption from these sites).

Related drugs
- Bupivacaine, prilocaine, ropivacaine (all are purely local anaesthetics)

Neostigmine

Class: Anticholinesterase

Indications
- Reversal of non-depolarizing muscle relaxants
- Myasthenia gravis

Mechanism of action
- Neostigmine inhibits the enzyme acetylcholinesterase in the synaptic cleft of neuromuscular junctions. This leads to a build-up of acetylcholine in the synaptic cleft and causes the desired cholinergic effects by enhancing neurotransmission.

Adverse effects
- *Common*: abdominal cramps, hypersalivation, bradycardia, sweating (all due to excessive cholinergic effects)
- *Rare*: muscle cramps, muscle twitching, rash

Contraindications
- Intestinal obstruction
- Urinary obstruction

Interactions
- *Aminoglycosides*: aminoglycosides decrease the effect of neostigmine
- *Clindamycin*: clindamycin decreases the effect of neostigmine

Route of administration
- Oral, IM or subcutaneous (all for myasthenia gravis), IV (for reversal of non-depolarizing muscle relaxants)

Note
- Neostigmine has a short duration of action (2–6 hours).
- Adverse effects of neostigmine can be antagonized with an antimuscarinic agent (e.g. atropine or glycopyrronium).
- Signs of overdose include abdominal discomfort, bronchial secretions, involuntary defecation and sweating.
- Neostigmine does not cross the blood–brain barrier and hence has negligible central effects.

Related drugs
- Distigmine, edrophonium, pyridostigmine

Nitrous oxide

Class: Inhalational agent

Indications
- Maintenance of anaesthesia (in combination with inhalational anaesthetic agents)
- Analgesia without loss of consciousness (e.g. in labour)
- Conscious sedation (especially in children)

Mechanism of action
- Nitrous oxide acts as a non-volatile carrier gas for inhalational anaesthetic agents.
- When used for analgesia in the form of an inhalational mixture with oxygen, low blood solubility of nitrous oxide leads to rapid induction and recovery with little effect on the cardiovascular or respiratory systems.

Adverse effects
- *Rare*: bone marrow suppression (following prolonged exposure)

Contraindications
- Pneumothorax (air pockets in closed spaces may expand)

Interactions
- None

Route of administration
- Inhalation

Note
- For analgesia during labour, nitrous oxide is used as a mixture of 50% oxygen and 50% nitrous oxide. This can be employed as patient-controlled analgesia (PCA).
- Nitrous oxide is not effective enough to be used on its own in surgery, but is widely used for general anaesthesia in combination with other agents (e.g. isoflurane).

Propofol

Class: Intravenous anaesthetic agent

Indications
- Induction of anaesthesia
- Total intravenous anaesthesia (TIVA)
- Sedation during diagnostic and surgical procedures
- Sedation during intensive care

Mechanism of action
- Exact mechanism is not fully understood.
- There is evidence to suggest that propofol may act on sodium channels in neuronal membranes.

Adverse effects
- *Common*: hypotension, pain on injection, tremor
- *Rare*: anaphylaxis, convulsions, respiratory depression, bradycardia, laryngospasm, delayed recovery

Contraindications
- Propofol allergy

Interactions
- *ACE inhibitors*: ACE inhibitors enhance the hypotensive effect of propofol
- *β blockers*: β blockers enhance the hypotensive effect of propofol
- *Calcium channel blockers*: calcium channel blockers enhance the hypotensive effect of propofol
- *Neuroleptics*: neuroleptics enhance the hypotensive effects of propofol

Route of administration
- IV

Note
- Propofol is widely used due to rapid recovery rate without nausea and 'hangover' effect.
- Slow administration is recommended in the elderly and hypertensive patients, as a marked decrease in blood pressure can occur with rapid administration.
- Propofol induces sleep in one arm–brain circulation time (3–5 seconds).
- The pain caused by IV injection can be reduced by giving lidocaine at the injection site prior to administration.

POISONING AND OVERDOSE

Many substances can be life threatening in overdose. An outline of the general management is shown below, followed by a guideline to specific treatments.

GENERAL PRINCIPLES
- Decrease absorption of the substance (by inducing vomiting, performing gastric lavage or whole bowel irrigation, or giving activated charcoal)
- Increase elimination of the substance (e.g. by forced alkaline diuresis or haemodialysis)
- Give antidote if substance is known

GENERAL MANAGEMENT
- Resuscitate the patient (**A**irway, **B**reathing, **C**irculation)
- Make every attempt to obtain a history (what, when, how much and route of exposure)
- Perform physical examination (if appropriate)
- If the substance is known, follow specific management as shown below
- If the substance is not known, blood and urine samples should be taken for toxicology screen and 4-hourly paracetamol and salicylate levels should be taken
- Treat any complications (e.g. dysrhythmia, hypoxia, hypotension, convulsions, hypothermia)
- Every patient should undergo a psychiatric assessment once recovered

Management of some common specific overdoses/poisons

ASPIRIN
- Measure plasma salicylate levels
- Perform gastric lavage if within 4 hours of ingestion
- Give repeated activated charcoal
- Replace fluid and electrolyte losses
- In severe overdose consider IV sodium bicarbonate (to achieve forced alkaline diuresis) or haemodialysis

PARACETAMOL
- Perform gastric lavage if within 2 hours of ingestion
- Measure plasma paracetamol levels (if at least 4 hours have elapsed since ingestion) and plot on nomogram
- If levels are in toxic range, give IV *N*-acetylcysteine infusion (if within 24 hours of ingestion) or alternatively give oral methionine (if within 10–12 hours of ingestion)
- Monitor LFTs, INR and U&E

TRICYCLIC ANTIDEPRESSANTS
- Perform gastric lavage if within 4 hours of ingestion
- Give activated charcoal
- Attach cardiac monitor and monitor acid–base status and ventilation
- Treat any associated complications (e.g. convulsions, cardiac dysrhythmias)

BENZODIAZEPINES
- Supportive therapy usually suffices
- Flumazenil (a benzodiazepine antagonist) is only indicated for rare, life-threatening overdoses, i.e. respiratory arrest

OPIATES
- Give IV or IM naloxone (a short-acting opioid antagonist)

IRON
- Perform gastric lavage
- Give IV or IM desferrioxamine

DIGOXIN
- Perform gastric lavage
- Give activated charcoal
- Correct any potassium disturbance
- Give digoxin-specific antibody in serious overdose

LITHIUM
- Perform gastric lavage
- Increase fluid intake to increase urine production

- Provide supportive treatment
- In serious overdose perform haemodialysis

CARBON MONOXIDE
- Give 100% oxygen
- Measure carboxyhaemoglobin levels
- Consider giving hyperbaric oxygen if carboxyhaemoglobin levels > 20%, if patient is pregnant, neurological symptoms are present or cardiac dysrhythmias occur

CYANIDE
- Give IV dicobalt edetate followed by IV dextrose

β BLOCKERS
- Give IV atropine for hypotension and dysrhythmias
- If this fails, give IV glucagon (to achieve a positive inotropic effect)

THEOPHYLLINE
- Perform gastric lavage (only within 2 hours of ingestion)
- Give repeated activated charcoal
- Correct any hypokalaemia with IV potassium chloride
- Cardiac monitoring is required (as there is a danger of dysrhythmias)
- Give IV diazepam for any associated convulsions
- *Note*: tachycardia, hyperglycaemia and hypokalaemia may be reversed with IV propranolol (contraindicated in asthmatics)

FURTHER READING

Aitken, J. M. *et al.* (1999). *British National Formulary.* 37th edn. British Medical Association, London.

Axford, J., ed. (1996). *Medicine.* Blackwell Science, Oxford.

Ballinger, A. & Patchett, S. (1995). *Pocket Essentials of Clinical Medicine.* W. B. Saunders, London.

Brown, A. F. T. (1996). *Accident and Emergency Diagnosis and Management.* 3rd edn. Butterworth Heinemann, Oxford.

Calvey, T. N. & Williams, N. E. (1997). *Principles and Practice of Pharmacology for Anaesthetists.* 3rd edn. Blackwell Science, Oxford.

Cass, N. & Cass, L. (1994). *Pharmacology for Anaesthetists.* Churchill Livingstone, Edinburgh.

Gilman, A. G., Hardman, J. G. & Limbird, L. E. (1996). *The Pharmacological Basis of Therapeutics.* 9th edn. McGraw-Hill, New York.

Grahame-Smith, D. G. & Aronson, J. K. (1992). *Oxford Textbook of Clinical Pharmacology and Drug Therapy.* 2nd edn. Oxford University Press, Oxford.

Hope, R. A. *et al.* (1998). *Oxford Handbook of Clinical Medicine.* 4th edn. Oxford University Press, Oxford.

Impey, L. (1999). *Obstetrics and Gynaecology.* Blackwell Science, Oxford.

Neal, M. J. (1997). *Medical Pharmacology at a Glance.* 3rd edn. Blackwell Science, Oxford.

Ritter, J., Lewis, L. D. & Mant, T. G. K. (1995). *A Textbook of Clinical Pharmacology.* 3rd edn. Arnold, London.

Sleigh, J. D. & Timbury, M. C. (1994). *Notes on Medical Bacteriology.* 4th edn. Churchill Livingstone, Edinburgh.

Stockley, I. H. (1994). *Drug Interactions.* 3rd edn. Blackwell Science, Oxford.

Waller, D. & Renwick, A. (1994). *Principles of Medical Pharmacology.* Baillière Tindall, London.

Winstanley, P. & Walley, T. (1998). *Pharmacology.* Churchill Livingstone, Edinburgh.

INDEX